FOR THOSE

with

EMPTY
ARMS

EMILY
HARRIS
ADAMS

FOR THOSE

with

EMPTY
ARMS

A COMPASSIONATE

VOICE FOR THOSE

EXPERIENCING

INFERTILITY

Familius books are available at special discounts for bulk purchases for sales
promotions, family, or corporate use. Special editions, including personalized covers, excerpts of existing books, or books with corporate logos, can be
created in large quantities for special needs. For more information, contact
Premium Sales at 559-876-2170 or email specialmarkets@familius.com.

Library of Congress Catalog-in-Publication Data

2014959241

Paperback ISBN 978-1-939629-60-9
Hardcover ISBN 978-1-942672-75-3
Ebook ISBN 978-1-942672-03-6

Printed in the United States of America

Edited by Brooke Jorden
Cover design by David Miles
Book design by Maggie Wickes

10 9 8 7 6 5 4 3 2 1

First Edition

CONTENTS

Here, I acknowledge the many people who have
helped me both shape and share my story:
my creative writing teachers, my family,
my fertility doctors, and most of all, my husband.

This book is for all those with outstretched arms.

May your arms one day be filled.

Introduction

$\mathscr{E}$ very fertility journey begins with a feeling of foreboding, an uneasy tickle that starts in both the mind and the womb. After seven months with no pregnancy, my husband and I began consulting physicians. Doctors asked questions ranging from how often we had sex to how much hair we grew—and where we grew it. They took nearly every bodily fluid imaginable for testing. For nearly a year, the results all said "normal."

Every day for months, I took my temperature in the morning to check for ovulation. Sometimes I fell asleep with the thermometer in my mouth; sometimes I waited, bladder nearly bursting, for the thermometer to register my temperature so I could get up to pee. Moving too much could skew my results for the day and ruin my entire month's chart.

For most questions, we needed to wait a month to get an answer. Every new cycle meant another answer and another failure. I knew something wasn't right, but that didn't make hearing "The Answer" (the answer that told us the real problem behind our childlessness) any easier.

By the time The Answer came, I knew a lot about infertility and what could go wrong. I knew about oligospermia and endometriosis, about PCOS and Rh incompatibility. I knew, in an intellectual way, that our infertility could be caused by a disastrous bodily malfunction. But I didn't expect our situation to be dire. Not even at the doctor's office on that horrible day.

I sat with my husband on my right side—between me and the exam table. We were waiting for test results. Beside me and to my left stood a desk with a little model of a womb, donkey-eared and flabby looking. I preferred the little womb to the exam table and its much-hated stirrups. I remember wondering how many more times I would be forced to stick my feet in those before we could get pregnant. Three? Four?

When the doctor came in, I could tell this time the test had revealed the problem. My mind grasped at a few possibilities: bad cervical mucus, maybe my pH level was too high, or maybe a bit of tissue needed to be cut away. The doctor paused at the door, taking a last moment to compose himself. In that moment before he told us the results, I felt a blooming excitement. If we understood the problem, I thought, we could fix it. Until then, we'd only found out what *wasn't* wrong. Now, I thought, we could move forward.

When the doctor explained what he'd found, I understood the implications. It meant the possibility of no biological children. Ever. I sat there and listened, and then I wanted the doctor to leave. I wanted him out. I felt guilt and anger wanting to take over. Guilt, because the betrayal came from our own bodies, so it must be our fault. Anger, because all the time and effort and stirrups might have been for nothing.

I wanted to give in—react to the news, and react in private. Later, I would feel lonely in my crisis. I would want to know that other people knew and understood the depth and breadth of my pain. However, when The Answer first came, I wanted everyone but me and my husband to just disappear. I wanted solitude. If my husband and I could just be alone, it wouldn't matter if we could or could not get pregnant. If we were alone in the world, we could just let the grief take over. I wanted isolation.

But the doctor didn't leave. Not until after giving some advice on what to do next. I felt like the world outside must be flaking away into insignificant bits. The only events and people that could possibly matter sat talking in that room. The rest might face the imagined apocalypse outside without my noticing or caring.

But when my husband and I left the office, the world did not reflect my post-apocalyptic expectations. Normal-looking people sat in the lobby. The streets were still paved and cars still drove on them. The world had ended, but then, with inexplicable speed and accuracy, it had rebuilt itself. Except for me and my husband. Everything else was remade, perfected even. Except us.

For a few months afterwards, my husband and I spent our time fluctuating between the normalcy of our life before and the deep hopelessness of the new. I found I could still participate in activities I'd always enjoyed. I still wrote poems. I still baked cakes and cookies. But the frustrations of pre-infertility life morphed under the pressures of post-diagnosis life, becoming catastrophes. Cleaning the toilet made me cry. I needed a nap after editing my technical writing. Sometimes I just sat down and refused to do anything.

I watched my husband change before my eyes. Instead of

letting out thunder-like peals of laughter, he stood quiet. Instead of telling animated stories, he sat back in his chair, looking at nothing in particular. In group settings, he often didn't speak unless spoken to.

We both exhibited physical symptoms of despair. I needed to rub Trent's back at night for him to be able to sleep. He needed to rub mine to get me to wake up in the morning. My stomach began to churn with a constant, dull ache. He started to grind his teeth at night. Both of us felt constant emotional fatigue. For a while, we didn't have the energy to even try to fix our emotional distress.

When I started looking for help, I turned to a source where I'd often found comfort before: books. I went to a local bookstore carrying a list of a few titles and authors' names. I found an entire bookshelf dedicated to pregnancy and childbirth, but I didn't find a single book about infertility. I asked one of the employees if he could look up the names of the books I'd brought. Handing over that paper felt like a moment of confession. The man saw the titles and, bless him, said nothing. He checked, but they didn't carry any of those books. He asked if I wanted to do a special order. By then, I felt so embarrassed, I just told him no and left.

I've been back to that bookstore in recent years, and they do sell a few infertility titles now, which makes me glad. At the time, I remember thinking: this should never happen to someone else. I don't want anyone else to come looking for help and come away empty-handed and alone. I knew then that I wanted to write about infertility, but I didn't know what to say. I didn't even know what I needed to hear, not yet.

When I did find books at the local library, I didn't react to them quite how I expected. I felt frustrated because they gave me information I often heard from my doctors and from medical reading: infertility is a common problem, there are many different treatment plans available, make sure you choose a fertility clinic you like. They were all valid points. But it felt like sitting through yet another infertility consultation. We already knew some of the statistics regarding the frequency of infertility. Every doctor's visit brought us deeper into our treatment plan. We felt comfortable with the specialist who treated us. I needed an indefinable something else. I needed something more than factual analysis. The repeated realities seemed to pile up in my mind, like a stack of brooms with no dust pans—useful in themselves, but lacking an essential element. I'm sure those books are a great comfort to many people; but for me, I felt frustrated with the fact that I still ached with an undefinable, unmet need.

What finally did help me feel less alone and more at peace was reading personal essays, short stories, and poems about infertility. I found them in women's blogs and magazines. I saw myself in these women who were willing to put their own experience down into words. While most of their stories varied from mine in some instance or another and some of their emotional reactions were different, I felt like I'd found some solace. I'd found my sisters in suffering.

I could write a book filled with medical facts, pages of statistics, and detailed anatomic illustrations. It would be a useful book, and I am sure there is someone who would need it. People need those types of books because those books are like brooms—made to sweep up the broken pieces of a dream. But my book is not like a broom. It's more like a dust pan; it's a place to hold broken valuables before they are remade. In this book, I intend to share my own experiences, the pieces of me that broke and lay shattered on the floor. The stories will be shards of varying sizes and not necessarily put into chronological order, just like all things are when they've been collected into a dust pan. You will see even broken people can be rebuilt—not into what they were before, but into something else just as glorious. I want people to know, that no matter how broken they might feel, their scattered pieces are worth the effort—not only of gathering but also of holding, and rebuilding.

Though my husband and I still have times when it is hard to wake up and hard to sleep, when our teeth grind and our stomachs ache, both of us have found ways to continue on with life. Instead of fluctuating from the old life to the new one, we blended the two into one. We've been gathered, held, and are beginning that process of being rebuilt. Part of my new life, my new self, is the desire to help those that are struggling like me. I've written these poems and essays as a way to add my voice to the voices of the sisters who helped to hold me. I'm here, and I want to talk to you.

PART ONE

THE ANSWER

Heartbreak

I often feel divided into two selves. One is infinitely stalwart, practical, fearless—solid. The other is easily frightened, quick to cry, worried—tense. For many years, I called the first my Rational Self and the other my Irrational Self. But I think I've been wrong in calling them that. Over the past few years, I've come to understand the true nature of these two selves. My Irrational Self is Fear; my Rational Self is Faith.

My years of living and surviving in an imperfect world built up an unfaltering part of me that believes there is purpose in suffering, nobility in enduring, and life after death. Even during times of crisis, in my deepest self, I've felt a benevolent God directing my life towards a great purpose. I would mourn, yes, but never for long, and never with absolute despair.

When my grandfather died, even as I grieved, I knew that I would see him again. But the diagnosis, The Answer, meant mourning the loss of children who never lived, and I didn't understand what solace I could find. My mind could not fathom a heaven without my children. But how would they get there if I didn't bring them into the world first?

During my time at the university, I always felt in control of my destiny. If difficulties arose, I could fix them. If I struggled in a class, I could study harder and find a tutor. When I decided that I wanted to be a writer and not a singer, I changed my major from pre-music to English. I faced hardships but always felt strengthened by the encouragement of Faith. With that help, I came off conqueror. I felt so confident in my ability to work my way toward my goals—so confident in my ability to control my destiny—it never occurred to me that my plans for the future might be thwarted. Not until about a year after Trent and I started trying for children. With the diagnosis, my goal felt like it rested an insurmountable finger's length out of reach. I couldn't even get close enough to fight, let alone conquer. Worse, my goal was no longer as insignificant as a grade or even a career. Motherhood had always been my ultimate purpose and I felt powerless to achieve it.

When the doctor told my husband and me why we weren't getting pregnant, the two of us managed to hold our emotions back until we got home; then it was like we melted. I cried. He cried. And nothing could make us stop.

Faith told me the same things I'd always known in a voice strong and urgent as ever. It also cried right along with the rest of me. Always before this, Faith had been removed from the grieving process. Before this, Faith felt no pain; it gave comfort and consolation without any damage to itself. Always before this, my undamaged, unshaken, tearless Faith pulled me from my grief. Now, even the most faithful part of my soul shook with devastation.

And why shouldn't I feel such deep desolation? Both my husband and I knew we wanted to have children. We knew from the time we were children ourselves. Part of why my husband fell in love with me was that he knew I would make a wonderful mother. I fell in love with him in part because I knew he would be an excellent father. We had both chosen our separate careers because we believed they would be most conducive both to our happiness and to having a large family. The first question my husband asked me after I said yes to his proposal of marriage was how many children I wanted. We decided on six before we even announced our engagement to our families. Even before we could become parents, our lives revolved around bringing children into a safe and loving home.

With that plan threatened by our own bodies, we were thwarting ourselves. True, neither of us ever picked over a list of physical infirmities to select the perfect cocktail against fertility, nor did any of our previous life choices cause the damage blocking our path to parenthood. It didn't matter. Our lack of fault couldn't restrain our feelings of guilt and devastation.

I believe that there is a point where sadness causes physical damage. It creates a sickness as destructive as any fever. Day to day life became exhausting. I especially remember the dishes being a source of great fatigue. Just looking at them made me want to cry. Doing the dishes made me tired, hot, and angry. My anger always hid just under that prime layer of guilt, blistering and uncomfortable.

My husband, still a student, found his homework to be an insurmountable obstacle. Pencil in hand, he sat at the table for hours, writing, then erasing. He didn't get angry like I did. For me, the diagnosis had triggered a kind of fight-or-flight response, and I fought. My husband just got quiet.

The previous year, we had hosted game nights almost every week. We invited neighbors over for dinner. We were even asked to plan activities for our church congregation. The year of our infertility diagnosis, our social circle shrank drastically. We found it difficult to go out among friends who we felt sure must be happy. Their apparent comfort and our certain misery made a mortifying comparison.

In short, I believe we were experiencing despair. For the first time in my life, I felt like my suffering wouldn't end. To make things worse, it was torture to watch my husband give in to discouragement. My attempts to cheer him up, my efforts to show increased love, and my continued research into fertility treatment could not bring him the solace he craved. Even doing everything in my power to help, I failed to stop his descent into despair. I could offer comfort, but not a resolution to our problems. I felt powerless in so many ways. No, I felt infertile: unable to produce a child or a miracle to save my husband or even a cupboard of clean dishes. All of my united impotencies felt like accusations. I suffered a roiling guilt. Nothing I did made the infertility go away. Nothing I did made the pain go away, either. The guilt and the sadness often paralyzed me, sometimes in the middle of a task. My capacity seemed to shrink, and that made the guilt bubble ever hotter in my stomach.

As the months passed, I made valiant attempts at being happy. Sometimes I succeeded, passing a whole week without thinking about what was wrong in my life. There are some who might even be surprised to see how unhappy I sometimes felt. I tried so hard, not just to show a brave face, but to actually be as brave as I wanted to be. I didn't want to be angry. I didn't want to be sad. I wanted to want to do the dishes and clean the toilet.

When the sadness returned, so did my guilt. I felt like my expressions of sadness amounted to nothing more than whining at the universe, at life, and even at that benevolent God I love. Of course, my expressions of sadness amounted to much more than that, but even the mistaken thought that my grief might be just a tantrum made me feel ungrateful, selfish, even childish.

When we reached the utmost extreme in misery, my husband and I decided to talk to our church's minister and share our situation. We knew him. Trusted him. And we needed to hear someone other than a doctor tell us it would be okay. The minister listened to both of us together. Then he spoke to each of us alone. When my turn came, he asked how I felt about everything. I started by saying I felt like I was doing a little better than I had at first. Which was true. My times of happiness stretched longer every time I reached that longed-for state-of-being. Then, because the need to say it just seemed to burst out of me, I said, "But sometimes it's just hard."

As I tried to control my face and keep it from crumpling into tears, the minister just nodded.

"Well, that sounds about right," he said. "Facing infertility, that's not an easy problem."

He let me know I wasn't experiencing exaggerated grief. He reminded me that even Abraham and Sarah, Jacob and Rachel, Zacharias and Elizabeth, and many other faithful couples, when faced with these trials, struggled. God knew the depth of our plight and didn't expect me not to feel grief. I had made all these points myself when trying to comfort my husband, or even comfort myself. But to hear them from the minister felt like permission to struggle: to be fighting the good fight, but not be done yet. I felt relief settle on me like a mantle. My responsibility wasn't to be impervious to grief. My responsibility was, and is, to become a better person. Just like it was before I was aware of our infertility.

The grief didn't dissipate after that conversation. I still mourn the loss of a very dear dream. Rather, I grasped that God didn't expect me to transform into a minute-made saint. Saints take time to develop over years of struggle. Even during my most despairing moments, I had known it wasn't faithless to grieve, but I'd not yet understood that it wasn't faithless to still be grieving.

I let myself feel the sadness with no guilt. No guilt for the wiring of my body. No guilt for the fact that I can change nothing on my own. No guilt for my need to mourn. The loss of my guilt gave me a sort of small redemption. The semi-paralysis began to lift from my muscles as if I were being cured of emotional tetanus.

I still tried to fight against the sadness, and that fight helped me reach a good equilibrium. Rather than gaining instant, unrelenting optimism, I understood that sorrow means sorrow, not failure. I no longer thought of myself as a whiner, but as someone recovering from a physical and emotional injury. Sometimes it's just hard. Sometimes I don't know how things will ever be okay. Sometimes I cry into a suds-filled sink and leave the dishes unfinished. That's about right.

Heartbreak is not a sin.

Blame

*I*n a world of cause and effect, there is always some traceable line of why something is happening. Historians track the causes of wars. The FDA can find the source of a salmonella outbreak. Scientist can find the loose electrons that cause chemical reactions. Our doctors found the reason why we haven't been getting pregnant.

Not all couples get the luxury of knowing what causes their problem. Science is still imperfect at finding the answers to all questions. Still, even without concrete proof, fingers can be pointed. Whoever required concrete evidence to cast blame? For Trent and I, we found out who and what, if not quite why.

Before we knew the diagnosis, we each felt sure we were to blame. I told Trent I was sure it was me. Trent told me he feared it was him. Neither of us wanted to be the one who caused all this trouble and suffering. Neither of us wanted the other to feel guilty. One day I would be crying into Trent's chest and asking if he would still love me if I could never carry a baby. The next, Trent would clutch me to him and ask if I would still love him if he could never father a child.

We wanted to find the exact source of our problem because if we didn't know what was wrong, we couldn't fix it. We did not want to find the source of our problem because neither of us wanted to blame or be blamed. Since both of us wanted so badly to be parents, each of us feared our bodily weakness might destroy the dreams of the other.

As these feelings grew and deepened, Trent and I became aware of a frightening reality: our chance of becoming parents is not and never has been the only dream at stake. Marriages often crumble in the wake of fertility problems. Our marriage is strong. We've supported each other through years of poverty, forgiven each other for arguments, supported each other during times of long study hours, and encouraged each other during times of unemployment. Even through seasons of distress and grief, we never let those times make us question our love for each other. But the stresses associated with infertility hit us hard and unawares. Blame in particular, slapped at us with its love-curdling, mercy-pickling hand. Even love as strong as ours cannot survive prolonged exposure to the crippling weight of blame.

When The Answer came, we knew that neither of us wanted to blame the other, nor be blamed. Even with those desires clear in our minds, we did not know how to avoid those feelings. The reality of a diagnosis works like gravity, pulling the heaviest of emotions out of you. Then it pushes those feelings back at you like a repellent magnet. The resulting mess is that negative feelings push heavy on your soul even as they try to tear you apart. Your physical and emotional soul is in rebellion. The push and pull holds all the pain like a bruise just under the skin. It's so easy to react with even the slightest touch. We needed a plan of attack. The Horrible Answer came at us before we finished devising our plan. We were both thrown into a full-blown war against blame without a battle strategy.

We knew. We could both look at the diagnosis, black and white, indisputable. A nuclear bomb on a piece of paper. And we didn't know what to do. When I remember those first few months after the diagnosis, I see it as a time of gray. It's as if the good things, the colors, the instances of happiness, now lacked some element crucial to true joy.

We tried to be as good and loving a couple as always. But the blame we struggled not to give or feel made us uncomfortable. We each reassured the other that our love remained unchanged. We still went on dates. We still tried our best to make the other happy—putting the other's wants and needs before our own. Our efforts couldn't erase the horrible fact that we knew—we knew what, and we knew who. Neither of us bore any personal fault. It just was, and the knowledge burned.

The comforting words, the reassuring touches, and the absence of anger kept our situation from escalating, but it failed to resolve the deeper issue. The time came when the situation needed to be addressed head on. All our efforts toward removing blame from the situation came up as fruitless as a barren tree. We needed to know that neither of us blamed the other, but even more urgently, we needed a mechanism to make that acceptance, love, and understanding felt.

Since the early years of our marriage, our usual spot for difficult discussions is the bed. The tradition began in our first apartment, where we owned almost no furniture. To this day, when we need to discuss an important topic, we go to the bedroom, and on top of the covers, we cuddle close together to talk. The physical contact, the protective way we hold each other, the comfort of being warm and safe all create an environment ideal for discussing topics that make us feel hopeless. It reinforces that we are on the same team, even if we are struggling.

It is difficult to confess when we harbor hurt feelings—more so when both of us have been trying hard to avoid hurting each other. Despite the difficulty, we both acknowledged the tension each of us felt.

Partner #1, who received the diagnosis, felt the weight of the blame for our trouble, and that guilt proved not just crippling, but humiliating. Partner #1 felt the loss of so much money spent to fix things and the pain of so much emotional capital invested in a cure. The diagnosis only ensured the spending of more money and more emotional taxation.

Partner #2, who was diagnosed as "fertile enough," felt the other took too much credit for the emotional and financial hardships. Partner #2 felt helpless to ameliorate the situation. After all Partner #2's efforts, the reassuring words were not enough to keep Partner #1 from feeling the blame. Partner #2 worried that their love was insufficient to heal their partner.

You may notice two things from the paragraphs above. First, I mention that one of us is infertile, the other is fertile enough. Yes, neither of us is ideal in our fertility. It's quite common for one partner to be fertile enough, but not perfect. In most instances, that situation will go unnoticed. When paired with someone who is also less-than-perfectly fertile, you may or may not get a problem with conception. Paired with someone who is infertile, disaster can (and for us, did) happen. The second thing you will notice is that I am not saying who it is that got the worst diagnosis. The reason is this: we both got that diagnosis. I'll explain.

As we lay on that bed, we aired our grievances, but we also talked about how much we love each other. Neither of us regretted our decision to be married to each other. We reassured each other that even if we had known the extent of the troubles we would face together, we would still decide to be married. We are infertile. Not just one of us. *We* are. You see, we decided long ago that we share everything: money, furniture, books, cars, etc. We are a unit; everything we own is shared. On that bed, we decided that we would share the blame for this burden, too. We wouldn't choose to seek out a new partner, not even to become parents. We made the decision that we were committed to each other. We knew now that the decision to stay together meant it would be difficult for us to get pregnant.

We still must deal with the reality of the situation. One of us needs to go to receive treatment from the doctor more often than the other. One of us must claim the diagnosis on insurance forms. We both need to know that the diagnosis does not make either one of us think less of the other's qualifications to belong to their gender. Both men and women need to know that a diagnosis of infertility does not make them less of a man or woman, and each gender needs different forms of reassurance

We let the doctors take care of the separate flaws of our bodies. That's their job. Our job is to take care of each other, and we do so by uniting. We treat infertility itself as a single unit, the ailment of both partners together.

In this book, you will sometimes hear me refer to the situation alternately as "our infertility" or "my infertility." I use both terms, not because I am the one who received the diagnosis, nor because I am the one who did not receive the diagnosis. "Our infertility" refers to the fact that it will be difficult for us to get pregnant. "My infertility" refers to my own personal thoughts and feelings in reaction to "our infertility." Trent and I do not and will not hone the blame on either one of us, not even in this book.

The blame is ours; we own it like every other possession. We both take steps toward treatment. We try to go to every fertility appointment together, even when the other needs no tests taken and will not need to be there to help make new decisions. There is no individual blame. We made a decision to be husband and wife. We chose each other to be the parent of our children. We will be parents somehow, someway. With that kind of future, why should we blame each other?

Psalm of Not a Mother

God,
Save me from those quiet moments when I remember my
    disappointment.
Save me from the echoes of bad news, doctor reports,
uncomfortable silences; erase even the words of comfort.
Save me from the thoughts of what to do next:
of the pills to take, of the test strips to buy,
    and the temperatures to record.

Give me the clamor of everyday life:
the cacophony of the television, the thrumming of the car
    motor, the bustle of a house party,
the crash of glass needing to be swept, the roar of a
    lawnmower.
Fill my ears with the white noise of living.

Save me from the time unfilled by the needs of children.
Save me from the quiet to listen to the sounds that don't
    come from the nursery.
Save me from the leisure to think that something is
    terribly wrong.

PART TWO

THE

BEST-LAID

PLANS

Rooms

I often wonder about the significance of certain rooms. When I was a little girl, there was a room just off the entryway to our house. We called it the Front Room. Not the most imaginative of names. It held our piano—a beautiful, but badly-tuned upright—our movie collection, a couch with pull-out bed, and a host of family pictures. Most of the time, we used it as a way to get from the entryway to the kitchen or from the kitchen to the hallway on the other side of the entryway. On occasion we also used it as a place to host guests when they visited. I carry vivid memories of that space, but not from the times I grabbed a movie to watch, and not even from the time spent chatting with visiting family. I remember it for the times Dad and I would talk there.

Once every month, on a Sunday, Dad would take each kid aside for what he called an interview. During that interview, we told him about life, our concerns, our hopes and dreams. Not many grown men can sit and listen to the concerns of a four-year-old with absolute attention. Dad could. I remember telling

Dad about my loose teeth, my fears of the dark. As I grew older, my concerns changed to worries about the acceptance of my peers, questions about politics and religion, about what to study, and what career I would choose. The tradition continued into college, and when I came home for visits, I often found myself sitting next to Dad on the couch, talking for hours about my classes, my friends, and my dating life.

When I go home now, stepping into that place fills me with memories of the things I wanted and the secrets I told my father. It's a museum of childish hopes and fears. I can feel my siblings' dreams crowding mine, even feel my father's hopes for us. The space is so filled with what happened there, if my home disappeared, I would be able to find the missing Front Room just by the feel of the air.

It took years for me to find another room so filled with significance and purpose. As a college student, my life was largely vagabond-ish. I hopped from apartment to apartment, changing every school year. I stayed too little time to fill any apartment with much significance. Besides, not much living happened in the apartments themselves. I slept and cooked there, yes, but the real events happened in the classrooms, at the activities I went to with my roommates, and on the long walks to and from campus. When I left those places, I swept the walls bare of my meager decorations, emptied the cupboards, and left no trace of my eight months or so of existing in those tiny confines.

The only exception, the only living space that meant something to me in my young adult life, beyond being a refuge from weather, stood just off one of the main streets in my college town.

I still remember the little brick building of fifteen apartments. My cousin and I moved in together. The ancient shag carpet and the heavy oak wood cabinets reminded us of our grandmother's house. In this apartment, I started dating my husband.

Even now, driving past that place makes my head turn; I am called by the memories that waft from the brick like a sweet scent. It's a perfume made of pictures: of Trent and I kissing on deep, brown couches, of dancing barefoot on the carpet, of lingering goodbyes each night outside the door. The apartment is the birthplace of our romance.

When Trent and I married, we moved into a five-hundred-square-foot relic. The windows and doors leaked air and were dotted with dark mildew. In the kitchen, an old-fashioned milkman box opened to the outside. We kept our spare key in it. The hardwood floors, once fine, bore the gouges of innumerable couches, desks, and tables. The bedroom held our queen-sized bed, a dresser, and if we stood on our tip-toes, us. The bathtub looked twenty years old; the plumbing was decades older. On several occasions, the world-weary pipes vomited clods of rotting hair onto our feet as we showered.

We spent a short four months in that apartment, but I know it holds an echoing memory of us in it. If ever a person were to complain of its being haunted, they would say they heard the voice of a young couple laughing from the living room, the sound of the milkman door opening and the incongruous clink of keys. Too much living happened there, too much discovery of ourselves as people, too many hours spent becoming our own family for us not to leave an impression.

When we prepared to move, we tried to find a more modern, or at least less moldy, apartment. Living, as we did, in a university town, we enjoyed a few distinct advantages. The university provided low-cost dates. We attended lectures and concerts and dances. Everything we needed was close by, and we often walked to the market and our church building. The distinct disadvantage was this: a landlord can make three times the money renting to singles rather than married couples. Landlords with apartments for singles can charge per person, rather than by apartment. As weeks passed, we realized that most married housing was either too expensive, too far from our university, or too unavailable.

In desperation, I called the landlord of the apartment where I'd lived while dating Trent. Randy reminded me of my father, albeit ten years younger. He dressed the same, talked in almost the same rhythm, and even had similar eyes. Though I rented from him, I also considered him my friend. When I told him my predicament, he gave up quite a bit of money to help accommodate my husband and me. He rented the two bedroom apartment to us. As I filled out the lease, he expressed his curiosity on just one point.

"You know, there's a second bedroom," he said. "Are you planning on using it?"

Knowing that Randy cherished no major concerns for furniture nor which rooms saw much traffic, I understood the true and unasked question. Smiling, I whispered conspiratorially to him.

"We're hoping to need it sometime soon," I said, though

Trent and I still anticipated waiting another six months before even trying for children.

The second bedroom measured about half as large as the master. In my previous days of living in that apartment, I didn't spend much time in the second bedroom. I lived in the bigger room with my cousin, and even then I preferred to socialize in the living room or kitchen. As a single woman, I developed little emotional attachment to the second bedroom and fewer memories. Now, as a wife, the idea of filling that space with the scents of baby powder, formula, and (yes) diapers, made me feel giddy with anticipation.

We moved into the apartment after spending a summer living with Trent's parents. As we transferred our furniture into the place, we noticed a slight problem. The apartment already contained furnishing for three single people. We decided that, since the second bedroom would not be needed right away, we would put some of the excess furniture in there. We stuffed the three twin mattresses in the closet and, since it lacked doors, installed a set of long curtains to hide our makeshift attempt at tidying. A slightly unconventional fix for a very unconventional storage technique. Then we filled the room with the half-wanted artifacts from our first apartment: a self-assembled desk, a velvet floral-print couch, and a painting just pretty enough to warrant keeping, just ugly enough to match our couch.

Though maneuvering the furniture left us little breath for talking (and we used most of that breath trying to reason out how to fit three twin mattresses into an average-sized closet), we had enough air to make excited jokes about the room.

"When we bring our own kids to go to school here, we can tell them this is where Mommy lived when she was dating Daddy," said Trent.

"And then tell them it's also where they were conceived," I said.

"You know what they say about second bedrooms?"

"No, what?"

"They increase fertility!"

If only . . .

Never before did a spot fill with so much consequence before fulfilling its anticipated purpose. Always before this, a place gained significance after the accumulation of many endearing, purposeful memories. It's not that I would stare into the room and think about how it would soon be the place for Baby. Rather, when I needed to find a new place to put something, I couldn't put it in the second bedroom. It was as if an unacknowledged impediment rested somewhere in the back of my brain. The second bedroom already had a purpose. In my mind, the promise of a baby filled the room with too much future to hold any more present.

Our first year of living in the apartment must have been a lonely one for the second bedroom. We seldom went inside. We were too busy in the other areas in the apartment. We did homework in the master bedroom, where we kept our desks and computers. We cooked and ate in the kitchen/dining area, and we visited with friends in the living room.

We had waited a few months after moving in to start trying for children. During that time, all of our hopes then revolved around the master bedroom. I rarely looked toward the second bedroom. Even when the negative pregnancy tests began to pile up, it isn't as if I spent time worrying about filling it. No, it regained significance only after we found out we might never have children. A few weeks after that revelation, we moved my desk and my computer into the second bedroom.

It wasn't a momentous occasion where I decided, with self-conscious symbolism, that I would replace Baby with homework and writing. After the diagnosis, Trent slept in short, restless spurts. We both blamed his difficulty sleeping on the whirring noise from my desktop's fan. And so we moved the computer to the second bedroom—not out of helplessness, I might add. No, but the strange impediment in my mind had crumbled. There would be nothing else to fill the second bedroom with. Not for a long time. With its purpose as nursery postponed indefinitely, I could move my computer in.

As the months went on, and the fertility tests went on, and the time kept passing, and our hopes went unfulfilled, the second bedroom began to fill with junk. We moved a part of the deep, brown sofa set. We brought my sewing machine out of storage and put it on the self-assembled desk. The used textbooks we couldn't sell formed a pile in one of the corners; an old stand-fan stood (what else?) in the other. We stored the wrapping paper behind the couch. After rearranging our bedroom, we moved a dresser into the second bedroom. When I needed to do a hopping sort of dance to get to my computer, I instituted a ban on any more additions. But even then, both Trent and I lacked the physical and emotional stamina to do more than halt the influx of the things we didn't want enough to look at, but couldn't throw away.

We lived in the apartment for two and a half years. When the time came to move, it took two weeks to sort our own furniture from the apartment furnishings, the important papers from the scrap papers, and the useful items from the rubbish, not to mention deep cleaning every corner. In the last few days of the preparations, my patience felt as thin as cheesecloth.

In that time of worn-out nerves, I started looking at the second bedroom again. The dressers and couches, the paintings and desks, the computer and the sewing machine made their slow disappearances, leaving dust and the occasional fly carcass. When the room lay empty and vacuumed, I stood inside, looking at the place where I had worked for over a year. Instead of memories of typing and reading and dancing around clutter, I heard a voice clear as day.

"You know, there's a second bedroom. Are you planning on using it?"

I took in a deep breath, holding in the air like a shield against the other voices. They came anyway, one of them my own.

And then tell them it's also where they were conceived.

You know what they say about second bedrooms?

No, what?

They increase fertility!

I turned and left. The bathrooms still needed cleaning. I didn't have time to consider those voices, so I left them to stay where they were. I could feel them starting to ferment in my mind. If I took them in, I would become drunk with regret. So

I blocked the words by scrubbing sinks, showers, toilets, and floors. As we finished cleaning each room, we closed the doors behind us. With the door to the second bedroom shut, I could keep the memories and the hopes and the disappointments locked in there, too. I kept them at bay until our last night.

Only the bed remained. Lying beside Trent in the almost empty apartment, I felt my breathing get deeper and start to catch. Trent must have felt it, too, because he rolled toward me and pulled me into his chest. I rested my head and breathed.

"Homesick already?" he asked.

"Yes and no," I said.

"What are you missing?"

I couldn't think of a single quantifiable object I missed. No. Instead, I mourned the loss of a possibility.

"Remember when we joked about telling our kids they were conceived in the same apartment I lived in when we were dating?"

I felt him nod.

"That's never going to happen," I said. "We're leaving, and we're not coming back."

I'd never broken my heart over a vulgar joke before. But I remember imagining the shocked look on our children's faces as Trent and I laughingly told them the scandalous tale. I mourned the loss of one of the few concrete images of our children's future. The second bedroom would never be filled, not in this apartment. And I mourned the loss of a possibility: a baby to fill the room, a romantic history, and the memory of three people loving each other, rather than just two.

We did leave that apartment. We never went back, but now I have a room in the corner of my mind. In it, there's a self-assembled desk, a velvet floral-print couch, and a painting just pretty enough to warrant keeping, just ugly enough to match our couch. I keep a corner of the room reserved for a crib. Neither crib nor room is empty. Both are filled with possibility.

PART THREE

BITTER
REFLECTIONS

Envy

My desire for a child is now more of a hunger than anything else. I can hear a rumbling in my soul. I want children with every whirring electron in my body, so much so that I wonder why I'm not magnetized. The powerful want, the ache that has become a need, can cause a warping of self so intense it sometimes changes how I see the world. Worse, it changes how I react to it. Even the emotional units of myself that make up a part of the patina on my soul can change.

When I was little, my parents taught me a skill they knew would help me to be a happier person for the rest of my life. They taught me to be happy for the success of others, even if that success came at the expense of my own. I think most people call it being a "good sport." The term makes sense to me, because I learned this lesson first in sports.

I joined my first soccer team at the age of five. Though young, I already knew that not everyone could be a winner. At the end of a match, I never shied away from asking who won. Other adults would wave their hands and insist that winning didn't matter.

"You played well, that's what matters."

"Both teams were really good."

I think they worried I might either be downtrodden in

defeat or overconfident in victory. I was five, so I can't say that their fears were unfounded. So much of the living that happens before turning five deals with learning to understand and control the physical world. The metaphysical world of emotions still remains wildly outside of a five-year-old's understanding—much less control.

I feel like all humans are born with both an innate desire for success and the mistaken idea that success is contingent upon someone else's failure. At the age of five, I hadn't learned to temper triumph or deal with failure. I didn't always know how to feel happy for someone else's success, especially because I still felt like they could only succeed if I failed.

My parents, unlike the others, felt no qualms telling me the exact score. Not because they thought I wouldn't experience disappointment at failure or triumph in achievement. Rather, they wanted me to learn how to process and control those two emotions early in life. Win or lose, they expected me to join a line of my teammates to go and congratulate the other team. I still remember running over and saying, "Good game. Good game. Good game," with robotic monotony, accompanied by a high five. If I was disappointed, my parents reminded me that I couldn't win all the time. I could try harder next time, but getting upset now wouldn't change the outcome. If I won, I needed to remember to be humble. The same lessons applied later during vocal competitions, debate tournaments, and dance recitals.

The situation became more complex when my siblings began to branch out into competitive events as well. As my siblings and I grew, our various talents began to bud. Of course, we were all very different, and I found that I lagged behind some of my younger siblings in certain talents. One of my sisters danced every style from ballet to hip hop. Another performed gymnastics with amazing ease. My younger brother proved to be an excellent strategist. I'm a mediocre dancer. It took me years to learn how to summersault. And I have never performed a three-move checkmate.

It is one thing to be happy for a stranger for a few moments. It's another to always be happy for someone who lives with you and who is consistent in their ability to outperform you. Of course, it did help that I have always loved them. It helped, too, that I began to see that my sibling's success didn't come at the expense of my failures. Their talents and successes, their weaknesses and failures, all developed independently from me and mine. I saw that jealousy never brought me any joy or improvement, and so, I made a conscious decision to experience more generous emotions.

Since reaching adulthood, I never considered myself to be an envious person. In fact, I know that, in general, I look at joyous moments as instruments to enhance everyone's general happiness. I find genuine happiness in the joy of others. I feel a little vicarious thrill when a friend gets a new job. Those engagement announcements with pink-filled joy make me giggle with delight. I go to plays where those I know are in the cast, and I watch for them whether they are playing the lead or dancing in the back of the chorus line. When someone announces their pregnancy, I . . .

I can remember the first time it hurt me to hear that another of my friends was pregnant. I remember her wearing a pink dress. It hung straight over her still-flat belly, but her hands were pressed over her stomach all the same. If I could sculpt, I would create a statue of her and name it "Bliss." I had been trying for over a year at the time. A few months earlier, my friend had told me that she and her husband would soon be trying for a child.

I still remember looking at her as she made the announcement, the odd feel of the muscles in my cheeks as I smiled—how they felt like strings tied to the corners of my lips. I congratulated her. And though I would never want to take away her happiness, I harbored a desperate desire to be pregnant, too. Sometimes I still remember that moment when I saw a pink dress. The recollection of the contrast between us still makes my fingers go cold. She, looking so happy. Me, feeling alone and unfortunate.

I went and sat down as soon as I could—wanting to get away from the dishwater mix of emotions that seemed to be roiling in my stomach. It was the first time it hurt me to hear a pregnancy announcement, but for all its newness, the pain pressed real and potent on my heart.

I didn't want to feel that way again. Ever. Though the sadness felt bad enough, the guilt felt even worse. Envy works like that—attacking you with a dual corrosiveness. First, it erodes the way you feel about others, then turns inward to eat away at how you feel about yourself. I worried that my friend might have seen a flicker of anguish on my face, maybe felt my yearning. She shouldn't need to spend her moment of happiness comforting me. Years have passed since that day. I lost touch with her long ago. She might not have seen the envy in my eyes. I know from experience how hard it is to see sadness when you yourself feel so content. Whether she saw or not, the moment passed without either of us saying anything to make the other uncomfortable.

I don't think I felt actual envy at this, my first moment of sadness. I think it's normal and harmless to feel sadness when someone reminds you of your trials—even if that reminder comes from simple contrast. The problem isn't the sadness; it's not even the comparison of "She has it and I don't." It's when you start to feel like you deserve the blessing more than someone else that the real problem starts.

Months, maybe even a year after my friend's announcement, I noticed my own slight pocket of festering emotion. On the Fourth of July, Trent and I joined my family for a firework show at a local park. During the hours before the fireworks began, we picnicked and played cards. The park had been crowded long before we got there, and the throng only grew more dense as showtime approached. It doesn't surprise me that it took me so long to notice the family sitting so close to us. In a crowd, it's hard to notice anyone.

When I did notice them, it was because of one of their daughters. I think she must have been sixteen or so. Like most people there, she wore a pair of shorts and a tank top, but unlike most other people, hers could not contain the great swell of her pregnancy. A few inches of fleshy belly protruded over the shorts. I stared at her and felt a deep clenching start in my own stomach. I fought the emotion down and tried to return to the card game. I didn't look at her, but I could still hear her.

She talked about how she wasn't sure about finishing high school.

"My boyfriend's got a job. He's got enough money. Why bother?"

She talked about the difficulties of alcohol and nicotine abstinence.

"I hate that I can't drink a beer. And geez, if you're gonna smoke in front of me, at least give me a puff."

I just sat there in horror.

The card game couldn't hold my attention anymore, and I found that I spent a good part of that Fourth of July with a family other than my own. I heard the brother talking about his recent stint in prison. I heard them chatting about smoking and drinking and drugs, and I felt an aching fury battling inside me.

She looked and behaved like some caricature of irresponsibility, deliberately placed just in front of me to torment me. I can't claim to be the patron saint of dietary excellence. I like diet sodas and French fries and the like, but I try. At the very least, I don't smoke, drink, or use recreational drugs. I also can't claim boundless wealth or vast stores of knowledge or any other absolute perfection. BUT. I have a reliable husband. Both he and I received a good education. We show promise in our careers of choice. My family and his are full of exceptional people. Though we aren't wealthy, we can offer a good home to a child. Here sat this girl who had none of those things, at least not as far as I could see.

The thought came to me, *She doesn't deserve "It."*

It. Meaning any of it: the pregnancy, the happy expectation, the baby, the chance to be a mother. It's a cruel, awful, horrible thought. I have no right to judge her. I spent a few, short hours' time near her. I never met her. Never saw her at home. Never saw into her heart. I know I have no right to pass any sort of judgment on her. I knew it was wrong then, too. But during those few hours, I didn't care enough to stop thinking about "It."

I thought all about my own strenuous efforts for a child: investing thousands of dollars, submitting to nurses poking me with countless needles, shoving my feet up in the stirrups so many times it made me want to scream. I had struggled so hard and expended so much hope, energy, and love for a still-absent child. And this girl across from me was making plans to be a mother. Not me.

In that moment, I recognized the envy buried deep in my heart. My sadness no longer sat dormant and harmless. Instead, an angry bitterness grew in its center. Discovering my flaw felt like finding a pocket of gangrene under just-healed stitches. The strength of my emotions shocked me just enough to wake me from my angry trance. I wanted to spend my time with family and enjoy the firework show. I shoved my resentment aside. Knowing I would need to address it later, I turned my attention back to my own family.

Sorting through my myriad emotions proved difficult. Concern for the child's welfare, that concern was legitimate. From what I saw, the child would be entering a home where no one put education as a priority and where questionable morals might make a significant impact on the child's life. But my concern, though powerful, occupied a lesser part of mind.

My first thought related only to this girl's worthiness for motherhood.

As I sat thinking, I tried to call up a single example of perfect motherhood and couldn't. I know of many laudable mothers. Some have even had angels come to announce their imminent pregnancy—proclaiming their highly favored status among women. But I can count the amount of recorded annunciation scenes on my hands.

If worthiness equaled fertility, what would that say about me? And didn't it hurt me to think that maybe there might be some who thought my lack of a child indicated a lack of worthiness? I didn't want to be judged. Shouldn't I give this girl the same courtesy?

I rehashed all the girl's imperfections. A part of me wanted to justify my envy. I couldn't recall a single person, other than this girl, who I felt didn't deserve their child. Still, I knew that this incident could prove to be a turning point. I could choose, here and now, if this would remain an isolated incident or if it would become a pattern of behavior. If I let this feeling run unchecked, my core self might one day mutate. Instead of feeling sadness for myself and happiness for my friends, I might shrivel into a bitter reflection of myself, always angry and aloof.

I knew I must find some way to harness my feelings. Envy destroys the soul. The thing is, I can't quench the desire to become a parent. That desire is a part of me. That need to be a mother is an ingrained part of my soul. To squash it down would be a betrayal of the goals that shaped my life since childhood. What's more, just deciding I don't want children will not help me achieve emotional happiness. If I decide to squash the desire to achieve my goals—even the impossible ones—eventually, I will wind up with no ambitions, no dreams. I feel like that would leave me an empty shell rather than a well-adjusted, envy-less woman. So, it's not the desire for children I need to quench; it's the negative feelings towards those who are going to have a child, while I am not.

One option is that I could just try to remove myself from situations where envy might become a problem. I could avoid baby showers and limit the time I spend with families with children. There are times when I decide to stay away from these circumstances. I have moments when I don't feel strong enough to face the sadness that can hit. I don't think it is bad to retreat from a situation that you feel unequal to facing. For me, however, I felt that the decision to always avoid such situations would not only be impractical, it would also be detrimental to my emotional health.

If I decided to leave the sphere of people with children, I could avoid confronting the issue, yes. I would also avoid the people I love. Most of my friends are parents; some have as many as five children. My husband is the second youngest in his family of six children, and as such, most of his older siblings are married with children. I've known and loved my nieces and nephews for years—some of them I've known since they were born. One of my sisters is expecting. I don't want to isolate myself from these people I love. Sometimes I struggle and feel very alone. I don't want to isolate the people who have always been my main support system.

Instead, I have tried to remember that my sadness is a separate thing from someone else's joy. It used to be that when I heard pregnancy announcements, I started to feel both the sadness for myself and the happiness for my friend at the same moment. Now, I try to hold the sadness off. I can feel the first stirrings of regret, but I send it someplace else, letting it know I will give it the attention it needs some other time. I let myself feel joy for my friend. It's real joy, not any type of falsehood or exaggeration. I can wait to take care of my regret until I have removed myself from the situation. With the sadness and joy coming at separate moments, I can take the time to remember that my sadness has nothing to do with the joy of my friends. They have made the decision to have a child quite independent of me. When I acknowledge that the pain is a trigger for sadness, but not the cause, when I remember that pregnancy isn't contingent on the mother's perfection, I can keep the envy at bay.

It Was the Bitterness

It was the bitterness,
the almost-silent purple pain
that lingered, gangrenous,
in the tissues of my heartstrings.

Each beat of lifeblood
surged through the poisoned veins,
taking a little of the rot as it flowed,
reaching to my uttermost
extremities, but causing most
damage to the little vessels
of the eyes, distorting the coloring
of my world.

PART FOUR

COMING TO
GRIPS

Nitty-Gritty

*Y*ou would think that after years and years of getting bad news, I'd be used to it. You'd think it felt a little different. It feels exactly the same: a moment of uneasy numbness—the same type of feeling that comes the first few seconds after a serious injury. There's no pain, per se, but the body knows that something disastrous has happened.

I take a few seconds to try to hang on to that numb feeling, not because I think I can hang on forever, but because I know that the news won't change. I want a few more seconds of life where I'm not obligated to feel that pain. I'm only in my twenties. I have decades of time to be sad. I'm a reactive person, though. My emotions come deep, hot, and fast.

I don't know if it's the same for everyone else, but I think my next emotion, after the numbness, is anger. It's a sort of aimless anger, not directed at any particular person, or even any particular force. I'm just angry. But I try to keep the same facial expression. I figure if I force my face into the emotion I want to feel, it will help. It never has yet. I don't know why I keep trying it. Sometimes, I say horrible, bitter things in this stage.

The anger starts to ebb, and in its wake, I feel helpless. I can't change bad news. I know it. The anger won't take away a diagnosis or a prognosis. I hate that. The inability to change my fate makes me feel small and childish. So I curl up small and start to cry. Crying doesn't help anything, but it does manage to make my nose plug and give me a nice, throbbing headache. That's why I associate headaches with sadness.

Then I start talking. I need to say something, anything at all, because words help me to process what I am feeling. I need to compare my experience with something I feel is more comprehensible. Poor Trent has heard so many metaphors come popping out of me in heartbroken sobs. Even after years of dealing with infertility, I still can't quite fathom the real depth of what is happening. I grasp the reality in an intellectual way. I understand what it all means. But my brain just can't hold on to it unless I paint a verbal reality for myself. Even still, there are times when I find myself sitting and wondering if I won't wake up from a rather long and vivid nightmare.

The initial process of grieving is always very much the same. The times that happen afterwards are worse, though. I don't talk about them too much in this book—not the moments when I hit rock bottom. It's not that they don't exist. It's not that I feel like no one should know. It's just that, most of the time, those are the moments when nothing happens.

When we got this new bit of bad news, I went through my usual routine of sadness. When I finished with the shock, anger, crying, and talking, it was nearly time for bed. We'd gotten the news in the late afternoon. I knew I couldn't go to sleep. My exhaustion made my head ache and my limbs sluggish, yes, but my mind kept whirring with unstoppable speed. Though I'm usually a morning shower-taker, I decided I would just take my shower for tomorrow that night. Trent crawled into bed. I started my shower, feeling awful. All the sensations from before were pulsing through me like emotive hot flashes. More than anything, the overwhelming reality of it all pressed down on me until I couldn't move. So I just sat down in the middle of the shower—not crying, just sitting. I sat there until I felt like I could go to bed. That is what I am like at rock bottom. I sit until I feel like I can move.

That's the nitty-gritty. Rock bottom isn't a place where there is weeping and wailing and gnashing of teeth. It's a place of nothing. Nothing happens. I can't write much about it because it would be about the way hot water keeps hitting my hair, about how time moves a lot like air currents if you sit still for long enough, and about how strange it is to come to yourself and realize that the only thing that has changed is that there's more to do and less time to do it. It's a still, but empty place. I don't like to go there, and though I think you need to know what it looks like, I wouldn't ever want to give you a lingering tour.

Reaching Okay

I'm okay—except for when I'm not. The times when I'm not cause a crippling effect similar to the emotional paralysis I felt in the early stages of our crisis. The results of those days are long stretches of time when nothing gets done. There are chores that need to be finished and bills that need to be paid. Not to mention the other projects I want to finish. I want to fill my days with activities, projects, and obligations that make me feel fulfilled, and even the things I enjoy have deadlines.

Which, by the way, is an amazing part of being okay: there are things worth waking up for. When I wake up in the morning, I don't feel disconnected or discontented. I don't feel cut off from the world or from my friends. I don't have the time, or the inclination, to always be sad. Frankly, I am done with being upset, overwhelmed, and unhappy. I am much happier being happy. So I am. Usually.

Just the other day, I found myself crying again. I'd been fine. Completely fine. In fact, I remember that day as a good day, on the whole. Trent and I went out to dinner with family. Then we all watched a movie. After chatting for a little while, Trent and I started home. We felt okay. More than okay, we felt happy.

After the usual bedtime routine of face washing and teeth brushing, we crawled into bed—where I started to cry. I couldn't believe that after months of not crying about infertility, I was sobbing into Trent's chest, his arms tight around me with bewildered concern.

The next morning, I could feel it again: that strange, almost headache-like feeling that starts at my eyebrows and sifts throughout the rest of my body. I felt the same all-encompassing disappointment that first hit several years ago. I didn't want to be awake that day. But I refused to go back to sleep. I got up.

You see, I'm fighting it. There's this horrible black pit I remember falling into during those first few months after Trent's and my diagnosis. I remember the condensed sadness that held me so tight in its embrace. It's full of short-tempered moments, unproductive days, sleepless nights, aching hearts, and acid-burned stomachs.

I'm fighting to stay out of the pit and in the real world. I refuse to go back, or at least I hope I refuse. The climb out takes so much effort, so much expended energy and time—time that I need to continue forward. I understand that there is a part of me that is still very uncertain about my future—that still feels afraid of the uncertainty ahead of me. It takes effort to move through the gloom ahead. In the fog, I can see stirrups, spent money, blood tests, and the sludge of possible disappointments. I can also see a little shape that looks like hope.

I'd rather go forward into the gray dawn than down into that black hole.

Okay

It is not to be unscathed
or unchanged.
It is to have once been un-undone.
It is to be put back together
in some functional order.
It is to be someone worthwhile,
even if you are someone different.
It is to exist in some frame of normalcy,
even if your frame of reference has changed.

PART FIVE

WHAT DREAMS MAY COME

Dreams

I have vivid, lingering dreams. When I was young, I would wake with my nightmares still coating my mind like oil. I would run to my parents' room and cuddle into their bed. The visits became so frequent, my mom developed a way for me to cope with the nightmares on my own. To save her and Dad from sleepless, loveless nights, she came up with an excellent idea:

"When you wake up, go back to sleep and change the ending of your dream."

I would wake panting, sweating, and with a remnant of the dream still in my head. Then, I'd go back to sleep and try to bend the dream to my will. It didn't always work, but most nights I slept long enough that the morning came before I could go back to my parents' room.

Most children outgrow their haunting dreams. I've known some adults who say they don't ever remember their dreams anymore. Mine became more intricate. I dream acid-like, plotless things that leave me with too bright images. I dream of sunshine-filled days of beaches with the deep black forms of whales under the waves. I dream of rolling across a snake mound over and over as the snakes leap from the many holes.

I mention the nightmares first because they cling to me the longest, but I have good dreams as well. Before my husband and

I were married, during the time he served a two-year religious mission, I would dream he was back at school with me. Before he'd left, we weren't even seriously dating. Even so, I would dream domestic dreams. In most of them, we were grocery shopping together. He would be there as I picked out lettuce and zucchini. I would wake up and expect Trent to be back and for new groceries to be in the fridge. The feeling would stay with me for up to ten minutes.

Trent's dreams are different. His pop like bubbles when he wakes. When the nightmares come for him, I simply touch his arm or rub his chest until he wakes. Sometimes, his eyes just flutter open; then he sinks back into a peaceful sleep. When I wake from a dark dream, Trent cuddles me for up to fifteen minutes, stroking my hair and whispering in my ear.

I don't like to wake him after a nightmare wakes me. If he wakes up and stays awake for longer than a few minutes, he struggles to get back to sleep. As the years of our marriage continue, I try more and more to bring myself back to reality after dreams. Sometimes, like I did as a child, I charge back into the dream and try to bend it to my will. Other times, I lay awake and repeat simple facts to myself, fighting off the lies of the dream. I stay still until I believe that all is well. It usually works. Unless I don't want to come back to reality.

One night as I lay asleep, I dreamed I was holding a baby in my arms. Her name was Mary Cook, and she was a twin. That's what it said on the birth certificate. She was maybe eighteen months old. Her hair was the amber shade of blond that I knew would one day darken to brown. I was holding her, her weight pressing into my hip. She didn't quite trust me yet. Her eyes regarded me in that assessing way only possible in infancy. I could see her open wariness in the downward thrust to her eyebrows and the index finger shoved into her mouth. I couldn't stop looking at her. As I stared, I noticed that her nose turned up at the tip.

"Your nose is just like Winnie the Pooh's," I said.

She frowned, not liking the name.

"Winnie the Pooh!" I said again, this time puffing the "p" sound, making her feathery hair poof around her.

She smiled: a tiny, reluctant smile, tugged sideways by the finger in her mouth. I knew then that she would love me, someday. I already loved her. Behind me, I could hear Trent playing with her twin brother. He laughed as Trent played with him. It didn't surprise me. Children often love Trent from the moment they see him.

These children were ours, or soon would be. The papers were sitting in front of us, only lacking a signature. We'd forgotten a pen, so we sat waiting for an adoption official to bring us one from an office. Mary's face started to pull back in to that distrusting scowl again. So, I started to bounce her on my hip.

"Pooh!" I said, with another puff.

She smiled again. I thought that maybe if I blew her hair one more time, she would start to laugh like her brother. I closed my eyes and started to blow. Instead of laughing, she shifted her weight toward me, and I knew without seeing her that she was coming in for a hug. I tried to pull her in close. My arms touched my own chest. I woke up.

I awoke to a dark room, which confused me. I remembered being in a room with bright, florescent lights—not here. I looked to Trent, expecting to see him holding Mary's brother. He was asleep next to me on the bed. A slow feeling of dread started in my chest and crept up my arms. I'd lost her. Without conscious thought, I plunged back into the dream. Without even completely realizing I had been asleep, I went back to try and bend the dream.

Trent and I were running, looking for them both. The lights were even brighter than I remembered. Scenery flickered in a distorted fashion. Distances seemed to change in strange ways, the scenes morphing in lurches. As the world shifted, I saw the two of them toddling away. I tried to speed up, and reached out my hand to scoop Mary back into my arms. I woke up instead. My heart pounded against my ribs, much too hard to let me sink back into sleep.

I sat up and looked around our bedroom. A small, heartbroken part of my mind started to realize it might have been a dream. Still, the panic did not go away. In retrospect, I think I preferred the panic to the heartbreak. I lay on the bed and thought hard. I didn't recall taking any steps toward adoption. But I had been holding her in my arms. I could still feel a warm spot over my right hip bone. Deep in my heart, I knew Trent and I wanted to try in vitro before we researched adoption. But I also had given her a nickname: Winnie the Pooh.

We were living with my parents for the summer; two months weren't enough time to be approved for, let alone selected for adoption. But I could remember seeing her adoption papers. I couldn't dredge up a single memory of completing paperwork, agreeing to a background check, or even walking into an adoption agency. But I had left her alone. Still confused, I got up and went to the computer in the next room.

I searched my email for any record of correspondence with an adoption agency. Nothing. I started an internet search for adoption agencies nearby. None of them looked familiar. Not a single one. I searched her name. Still nothing. I didn't even know what I could do to look for her. The functional part of my mind began to speak to me again. Other than this dream, I couldn't produce a single thread of physical (or even metaphysical) evidence that Mary Cook existed. It must have been a dream. I could think of no other explanation.

As I stared at the computer screen, my fingers slowed to a stop on the keyboard. I rebelled against logic. Taking a sticky note, I wrote down the name. *Mary Cook.* I'd already forgotten her brother's name. That thought made me shake on the inside. Still, some part of my half-asleep self thought, *He was Trent's responsibility. Trent was holding the little boy, not me. Trent will remember his name.* I took the paper back to my bedroom and set it on my nightstand. Trent still lay there, asleep. I knew I could never get back to sleep with so much adrenaline in my system. Not wanting to wake him, but not wanting to be alone, I crawled under the covers, waiting.

I've seen mothers in the supermarket panic over lost children. They start walking and softly calling their child's name. I've seen their pace increase, minute by minute. I've heard their voices get louder and higher in pitch. Now, I felt like that mother, except I wasn't even in the same building where I'd last seen my children. I had nowhere to search, no child to hear me call. So I waited in a half state of panic for Trent to wake up.

By the time he woke, the dream still hovered in a faint nimbus around me. I felt almost certain it had been just a dream. Still, the faintest hope/dread/joy/horror/something in me whispered it might have been real. The clock read 7:30, over an hour past when I first woke. Never before had a dream lingered for so long.

I told Trent everything. I told him about the nameless twin boy, about the adoption papers and how we'd forgotten a pen. I told him about amber-blond hair and Winnie the Pooh. I told him about waking, going back to find her in my dream, waking up to try and find her here. I told him about waiting for him to wake up. I never saw any recognition in his eyes when I talked about the twins. He didn't know the name scribbled on the sticky note. When compared with my usual dream-trances, this amounted more to a haunting—appropriate, because I surely felt haunted.

"I looked," I said. "I couldn't find her."

"Oh, Honey," he said.

I felt him try to pull me in close, just like I had tried to pull Mary in. I couldn't bear it. I pushed him back.

"Did I abandon her?" I asked.

"No," he said, trying to soothe me. "You didn't abandon her. She was never real."

The dream burst. I thought the release from the dream world would bring relief. It didn't. Instead, I felt a cracking sensation run right down my sternum. I started to cry. Trent was right.

There had never been any adoption meetings. There had never been any papers to sign. She was never real. I'd left her all the same.

There Is No Death with This Blood

There is no death with this blood.
No, this blood is only a testament
of the life that didn't start.
I should not be mourning the loss
of a barely-imagined, only-hoped-for Her.
It's only that there were moments
I thought I sensed someone there:
when I envisioned
stubs of fingers forming on a blooming hand,
new eyes beginning to stretch still-sealed lids,
though I know it would have been far too early
for more than a sanguine division of cells.
This blood is not Hers; it's mine,
and it has been coating my womb,
not pulsing in my veins.
It's been still and pooling for nearly a month.
There was no violence, no struggle,
no sudden cessation of movement.
There is no death with this blood,
but She's gone all the same.

Walking on Water

Two nights ago, as I lay in bed,
I felt the mattress suddenly curve and harden
into a wooden boat.
The teary wetness on my face slid seamlessly to drench
the rest of my tired body.
The rough breath of the barely-crying left me in one great
    rush
and became the storm that tossed my feather-made vessel.
It happened with such fluid senselessness that I did not
    feel the slip
from waking to sleeping. I did not know I slept.
All I knew was I was on a boat,
in a storm. And I must get to the shore.
There were no oars. None.
And I knew I could not swim in the flesh-rending
water of the wind-stirred current.
I dipped my hands into the surge and tried to paddle
    myself to safety.
But the waves held more power than my arms.
I yelled in competition with the wind,
commanding its hurricane to stop, but felt only the words
    blown back
into my open mouth.
I held up my hands for God to take me,
but felt no returning grasp.
I would be lost; I knew it.
I saw the shore, but I could not get there.
Not in that boat.
With striking clarity, I thought of the one successful man
    to walk on water.
And I remembered the man who had tried and failed.

I thought of my own weight and how it should make me
   sink;
it should pull me under the waves,
and I knew that here in the boat, at least, I did not sink.
Oh God, I thought, *I do not want to sink.*
I cannot stay in the boat. And I do not know how to walk on
   water.
I stood. Crying. Terrified.
I stepped free of my floating trap.
And did not sink.
My weight balanced on the water—solid and cold as
   gelatinous ice.
In my exultation, I did not see the wave that slapped me
   off my feet
and sent me rolling on tops of the breakers.
I stood again and, gasping, fought against the violence
   beneath my feet.
Blinded by rainy wind,
battered by waves,
bruises bursting beneath my skin,
I walked toward my last sure glimpse of the shoreline.
Each shift of the water unbalanced me.
Each blast of sea-spray sucked warmth from my body.
Each moment was a battle to move forward.
But I was walking on water.
Oh God, I thought, *keep me above the waves.*
Keep me from falling too deeply.
I would not ask, but I could not have moved.
Not in that boat.
It was a fight toward the shore and in my mind
I wondered and hoped someone might shout, "Peace. Be
   still."
When no voice came, I wondered if maybe God wanted
   me to drown.

But I couldn't wonder too long, because hiking up
a fifteen-foot wave took my thoughts as well as my muscle
    and breath.
It took hours, I'm sure, before I felt the telltale signs of
    sinking:
a sense of thickness and heaviness in all my limbs,
and the inability to lift my toes.
I cried and prayed, sure that I was going under.
I cried out, "Lord, save me!"
just I as sank to my knees in the surf.
Slipping in water down to my waist, I screamed;
then I was jolted by something solid but shifting under my
    feet.
I heard an answering voice say, "See? Sand."
And I woke up, crusted with sweat and salt.
I walked to the bath tub and washed
my feet before I thought to check my toes for grit.

Waking Up

*O*n those days when I'm not obliged to wake to an alarm, my wake-up time is a process of incremental self-inventory. Usually, when I first wake up in the morning, it's my eyes I sense first. Gummy, sandy, or heavy, I can sense them before the rest of my body. Next, I feel the part of me that is pressing into the mattress: sometimes the sinuous line of my side; sometime the press of my chest, stomach, and thighs; and every now and then, the press of my shoulders, hips, and calves. I am eyes and body, nothing more.

I wake up in puzzle-piece increments, and I never come to full awareness until after I've put myself back together. I don't start moving until I remember something that I want to get done: make breakfast or clean the bathroom, write an essay or go to the grocery store. The sense of purpose, however small, pulls me the rest of the way out of my comfortable sleep.

There are, of course, some times when my awareness starts somewhere other than my eyes. The most frequent exception is that I wake up aware that I can't feel one of my arms. The shocking responsiveness in the rest of my body and the complete loss of any connection to my arm wrench me awake. I lie in bed, sucking on my numb fingers to try and get the blood flowing again. When a strange appendage that seems to be made of gauze appears where my arm used to be, I shake the limb until it returns to normal.

On one special occasion, just after Trent proposed to me, I woke up feeling like every nerve in my body ended on the ring finger of my left hand. Every part of me wanted to be near the epicenter, the focal point of the new promise between me and my love. I lay still while my younger sisters (we were staying with my family) lay in their beds asleep. Even when they began to stir, getting up to use the bathroom and change, I lay in bed, grinning.

When our fertility crisis hit, my wake-up pattern crashed right along with the rest of me. I still remember that first day waking up after we got The Answer. The hard knot of my eyebrows woke me up. They were drawn hard together. Next, I felt a hard rock of emotion, buried deep in the center of my brain. I felt my body echoing the roundness of that metal spot; I lay curled in around my stomach. I did not want to think about why I felt so different. I did not want to remember anything about the day before. I did not want to get out of bed.

When I did remember and I thought about the doctor's appointment from the day before, I felt knocked off balance. Nothing about me or Trent had changed. We had only been diagnosed as what we had always been. Still, the diagnosis itself made me feel transformed, or rather, mutated. I didn't want to be this new person. I knew that going back to sleep wouldn't change anything. I didn't care. No purpose felt like enough of a pull to get me out from under the covers.

I'd never really thought much about what a miraculous thing

it is to want to be awake. The morning after my doctor's appointment, I felt like a part of me had pickled itself—had shriveled and soured with the brine of my disappointment. My first thoughts coherent enough to be more than impressions were, *It's still true today. And since it's still true today, it will still be true tomorrow. And the day after that. How can I wake up to this new truth every day for the rest of my life?*

All those thousands of future infertile mornings piled up on top of my head. I felt the weight of them pushing me into the mattress. I did need to get something done that day, many things I'm sure. But such was the oppressive nature of that weight that I didn't remember anything other than my shock and anguish. A part of me felt rather sure that sleep was the only way I could get away from how awful I felt. My body wanted to fight off my sorrow the same way I would fight off a fever—with sleep. Still, my mind came to the conclusion that this listlessness was not the same as the healing rest I get when I'm sick. So, with a grunt of effort, I got up.

The shock will wear off, I thought. *It's hard now, but I'll just get used to it.*

It took me a week before my body began to relax, the bigger muscles unwinding and uncurling. My eyebrows still curved down hard, like they were trying to crush my nose. My mind still held on to its little ball of disappointment. But my body did stop scrunching up in mimicry of my face. I began to sleep stretched out again.

Time worked its usual magic on me. In time, my sleeping body integrated the knowledge of our diagnosis into my self-definition. I no longer woke up in a state of anguished shock. But time is not a sufficient healer all alone. Instead of returning to my normal routine, I started to wake up feeling my stomach first. On my upper-right side, just under my ribs, I could feel a round and fiery spot, almost like a three-inch ball bearing. I sometimes imagined myself rolling back and forth on that pinpoint spot of discomfort. After rolling around in morbid fascination of my stomach, I felt my shoulders, wrenched tight together and pinned up by my ears. I still remember the myriad mornings when Trent kneaded the knots from my shoulders before I could (or at least would) get out of bed.

Time heals shock, yes. It does not heal ruptured dreams. It doesn't gloss over disappointed hopes. My body reacted to the stress caused by the new knowledge. I saw right away what caused the cramps and knots in my shoulders. It took me over a year to find that the pain in my stomach was caused by stress-induced digestion troubles. The pains, though constant, were minor. I treated them with antacid and Tylenol and back-rubs. The Tylenol and antacid and backrubs worked their own healing powers. The painful spot burned with less intensity. My shoulders rarely kinked into the same, hard knots as they did in the beginning.

The apathy I treated by trying to find activities with deadlines and places I needed to be at by a certain time. Not many—at least not at first. Those early days especially left me with a drag on my energy. My capacity for action shrank. It took time and effort to find a schedule that helped me feel neither apathetic nor overwhelmed. There were times I failed in what I wanted to do because I overexerted myself. There were other times when I accomplished nothing at all because I didn't give myself enough tasks to build up a good momentum. In time, I started to wake up with my first awareness in my eyes again. The day came when I could feel like an almost-whole self before forcing myself out from under the covers.

I wish I could remember the day I started to be pulled from my bed, not just out of a need to do something, but from a desire to be awake and doing something. I just know that, at first, those days came in spurts. Some days, I wanted to get things done. Other days, I just knew I needed to get something done. So, I got out of bed.

Only in recent months has the spot in my stomach gone away. My shoulders still tense from time to time, but Trent has a lot of practice massaging them. Waking up now feels similar to how I used to feel. The things I want to get done look different. Sometimes, I wake up feeling my arm first—because it's wrapped around Trent's waist. The point of connection between us wakes me with more sweetness than an awareness of just me ever did.

It took time, action, and then time again. But now, the deep part of myself that loves to be awake has woken up itself.

Deus Ex Machina

I like to drop the phrase *Deus Ex Machina* from time to time. It makes me feel sophisticated. *Deus Ex Machina* can be loosely translated as "the god machine." The term refers to a miraculous resolution to difficult problems. It originates from ancient Greek literature. Playwrights and bards often told tales where the gods would sweep down from the sky and rescue the hero or heroine from certain death/dismemberment/dishonor. You can see the trope used in every genre of fiction. In detective shows, a mysterious witness comes with a packet of uncrackable, court-admissible evidence. In fantasy stories, an all-powerful wizard chants an unbreakable spell, giving the hero new powers at just the right moment.

Sometimes I feel like I see my own future baby as my personal *Deus Ex Machina*. When I can't stand the pain of infertility a moment longer, I will conceive, or be selected to be an adoptive parent. *Once that baby comes, I think, the pain will dissolve like sugar in tea—lingering as a flavor, but not as a visible, touchable part of life.* Never again will I go to the doctor's office and worry about fertility, because I attained the long-sought goal: a baby.

But a baby is neither a god nor a machine. A baby is a being in need of a guardian capable of godlike love and machine-like stamina. When I sit and really think about it, I realize: I have been looking at this situation the wrong way around. I have been waiting for a child, yes. But my baby has also been waiting for a mother. And so it is that I, as a long-expecting mother, need to come to a realization: My children are not coming to save me. I am offering myself up to save them. Though I am far from godlike in my abilities, and though I have limited stamina, my child will not be my Deus Ex Machina. I will be theirs.

To the Son I Am Waiting For

To the son I am waiting for,
I have a dozen names picked out:
pressed, polished, and waiting for you
to come and choose from.

I have kept my hands scrubbed
and lotioned so they will be
soft when first I hold you.

I have kept my lips pursed
in a constant kiss
so they will be ready
to caress your forehead.

I have made you a thick blanket
of my arms so that you will never
be cold.

I have built a place for you in my heart
so that never in your life
will you want for a place to be loved.

To the son I am waiting for,
I want you to know, no matter how long the wait,
I will always be here,
so you will never arrive alone.

Until the day I see you, I am always,
your mother.

PART SIX

A MOMENT
TO RECOVER

Healing

$\mathcal{D}$uring fertility treatment, the concept of healing is an obsessively sought-for goal, but treatment lacks the same hurried pace as other ailments. The timetables are preset by the body to discourage sudden change. Even doctors and patients who hurry can only move to the slow rhythms of the body. Healing and treatment must be judged month by month, not day by day, much less hour by hour. After a month, you're either broken or whole. If broken, broken for another month at least. If whole, still uncertain about remaining whole until after a successful nine months pass.

Physical healing is more than fickle for those suffering infertility. Sometimes the cure comes before a treatment can even be chosen. On a random day, the body lets go of some unspoken inhibition and conceives. Sometimes healing comes and retracts itself. There is a child; then there isn't. Miscarriages and stillborn children shatter hearts that were only battered before. Sometimes the body taunts the sufferers with its own perfection. Nothing is wrong. But still no child comes. In some bizarre cases, the body behaves as if it has conceived when no conception occurred. Morning sickness comes, the belly swells: large and empty.

Infertility isn't like the common cold, where you can let

yourself be miserable until you're well again. With infertility, you must learn to be well, independent of healing.

Healing Prayer

God, grant me another day
of getting better,
another step towards
recovery.
Grant me the perspective
to see the changes for the better,
and the mettle to overcome
the inevitable steps backward.
Help the steps forward
outnumber those backward steps.
And if I'm destined to lose
ground, or even
to stay fixed in one place,
help me learn to live
in my new home.

Waiting

I finally left my spot on the road
where I waited for you for so long.
I left the little footholes where I dug
my heels and toes into the sandstone dust.

With little explanation, I took up my bed and walked.
Some of my fellows, the other Patient Faithful,
scoffed at my abrupt departure.
Still, I never turned into a pillar of salt.
Their calls never made me look back.
I was protected by inked-in words.
You see, I read while I waited:
memorizing the stories of those who found you
and of those who were left behind.

Of all the times you were found:
on the road to Damascus,
on the highway to Erfurt,
on the path to Walden Pond
you met your friends as fellow travelers.

PART SEVEN

PRACTICAL
REALITIES

Words

I am not simply a consumer of words. I produce them. In times of trouble, they are an antiseptic spread, an intravenous painkiller, and a powerful antibiotic. In times of joy, they are aromatherapy, herbal teas, and candied ginger. When experiencing times of extreme emotion, words pour from my mouth or roll from my writing fingers. I need to talk, to write, to express. Though I can hold words in for a long time, though I can let them bounce around in my head, though I can edit them in my mind for weeks on end, I need to let them out at some point.

People, in general, are loving creators and consumers of words. We open our ears to their sounds through radio and television. We read books. We attend the theater. We go to the opera. We consume words of all varieties, quantities, and qualities. Songwriters, poets, playwrights, screenwriters, and novelists produce more words than can be read or heard in a lifetime, but more and more still enter the trade every day. And because we cannot satisfy ourselves with commercially produced words, we solicit more. We ask questions.

The night of Trent's and my wedding reception, my four-year-old nephew asked me a question. The party was over; we'd all gone home, and I sat on a couch in my wedding dress, waiting for Trent to come and help me get back into normal clothes. The rest of the family was helping unload presents from the car. My nephew, still in miniature suit and bow tie, left the present-gathering in the hall to sit next to me instead. I love the utter guilelessness of children. I love how forthright they are with questions. Most of all, I love that they have not yet developed the idea that a question might be taboo.

Just hours after celebrating my marriage to Trent, my feet still aching from my wedding shoes, my nephew said, "Are you going to have kids soon? I want another cousin to play with."

He stared at me with such wide, eager eyes—completely innocent. At first, I started, feeling taken aback. Then, I began to laugh a little. I can still remember the feel of my slightly shaking ribs hitting against the dress's inner corset. Fighting not to let him hear my giggles, I tried to give a charitable reply.

"Oh, you want another cousin? Well, would you prefer a girl or a boy?"

He considered. "A boy, please."

"I'll see what I can do," I promised.

It was still a year before Trent and I began trying. Even with that time barrier in place, I felt happiness bubble up in me at the thought that I would one day bear children. I looked forward to having my kids play with my nieces and nephews, felt glad that they would have friends when they came into the world.

During the first year of marriage, not many people ask questions about children. Most seem to feel that a couple deserves a few months to figure things out. Besides, with pregnancy taking around five months for a woman to start to show, I wonder if some people are afraid of spoiling an announcement. And so, for that year, I remained safe from prying questions.

In fact, I brought the subject up again before anyone else. My sister Jessica and I attended the same university. On a walk between Biology and English class, I told her that I had three months of birth control pills left, and I didn't plan on renewing the prescription.

Many people weigh words by their quantity. A five-hundred-page book is of more value than a one-hundred-page book, for example. Of course, they are wrong. Words carry their own individual weight, which changes based on context. Over the course of growing up, my sister and I have exchanged thousands, if not millions, of words. Some of the weightiest and best we've ever shared came in that five minute talk across campus. I could feel that weight settle over me like a down coat: warm and immense. I expected to share even heavier, happier words later that same year. I never did.

Instead, Trent and I heard heavy words from a doctor, but these words fell like anvils on our backs: crushing and awkward to carry. As I listened, I knew for certain I didn't want anyone in the world to ever know that Trent and I carried such a weighty, embarrassing burden.

Of course, we told a few people: Our parents. A few other family members. But talking no longer held the same joy as before. We weren't sharing news, we were sharing statistics. We became soothsayers rather than conversationalists. We tried to throw out words of hope—for our benefit, sure, but also for the benefit of our beloved audience. It didn't stop the anvil from crushing either us or our loved ones.

I kept any unnecessary words bottled up inside me. Talking about the future—about children, about pregnancy and childbirth—no longer felt like candied ginger or herbal tea, much less like morphine. It felt like drinking saline solution. So I tried not to talk about it. Still, the need for words runs rampant, and so do questions. Those questions didn't come in a sudden flood. The taboo of asking about children wears off like a radioactive half-life. Most questions were simple, harmless, and easy to respond to.

"Any kids yet?"

"No, not yet."

It took two years of marriage before people began to ask why.

At first, I tried evasive tactics, vague answers about how timing is so hard to get right. Those answers don't hold up very long, and so the follow-up questions began to come in lakeshore waves: small but incessant.

"Are you waiting to finish school?"

"Not enough money, huh?"

"Waiting for a little more permanence in life?"

"Still getting to know each other?"

"Wanting to have a little more fun before kids?"

Still, I tried to evade a direct answer by shrugging, by changing the subject, or even laughing. After a while, I got sick of dodging. Instead, I said yes to everything because, really, it was all of the above. After graduation, it would be easier for us to seek treatment. We often did not have enough money to pay for expensive treatments. After getting more permanent housing, we might be better able to stay longer with one doctor. We knew each other's personalities pretty well, but both of us needed to find out more about the medical imperfections of our bodies. And of course, we would like to be able to have the fun that our worries often blocked. Yes. It all amounted to the same thing: no children.

Most questions simply caused mild discomfort and annoyance, and often came from people I did not want to be annoyed with. They just wanted to know more about my life. If all had been going well, I would have been more open. At least, I think I would. I'm under no obligation to answer questions about when or whether I have children. The persistence caused both Trent and I some discomfort and sometimes annoyance. But I am sure that most of these inquiries held no malicious intent. Despite times when I felt embarrassed or annoyed or upset, I could brush the encounters off. Usually.

One day, we were at a gathering of friends and family. For most of the party, Trent and I mingled together, but at one point, Trent went to get us both some lemonade. It's bad to be alone when you want to fend off questions, especially when in the proximity of a long-loved friend of the family. We had already handled a few questions about children. Even though we fielded those questions with success, my nerves were a little tender. Successful blocks still cause pain.

"So, when are you going to start your family?" she asked.

The question wasn't unusual, nor was the wording. In fact, I'd heard the question phrased exactly that way before. But my tender nerves couldn't take any more questioning. Already sensitive and a little upset, I felt my back straighten and my shoulders draw up. I did not want to be angry, not with this person I loved. Neither did I want to share the extent of our troubles. The freshness of our pain held me back from speaking. I thought telling her might just make me unravel.

"I have no idea," I said, voice as stiff as barbed wire.

Trent returned with the lemonade just then, and his arrival prompted a change in subject. I just listened during the rest of the conversation, not up to talking. Simple though the exchange had been, I felt irritated and uncomfortable. It was like my brain was filled with immovable, emotional itch weed.

On the way home, I relayed the conversation to Trent. As I mentioned the word *family*, my throat started to tighten, forcing me to clear my throat. Trent took a hand from the wheel and, without looking away from the road, took mine.

Waiting until he could stop and look at me, he said, "Next time someone asks you that, give them the date of our wedding. We don't have children yet, but we've been a family for years."

When our friend asked about "starting a family," she meant no reproach. If we had announced we were having troubles, she never would have asked when we would start our family. I might have saved myself some grief in that respect. But just admitting our troubles felt gut-wrenchingly painful. And besides, Trent's eloquent comfort eased an unrealized fear. His assuring words let me know he already thought of us as a family. We are a family, and have been for years.

Not all questions are so benign, though. And not all questions lead to transcendent moments with my spouse. Another encounter happened during a visit with my parents. We all went to church as a family. It was summer time, so many of the college students like me were also visiting home. I could see many childhood friends lining the pews. Between services, I noticed my mother talking to a young man a few years older than me. I knew him by sight more than anything. I went to join Mom.

Smiling, he held out his hand to shake.

"Hey, you sure grew up. I hear you're married now."

I smiled and shook his hand.

"Yeah, I am. I heard the same about you."

"I also hear you're twenty-four and don't have any kids yet."

It was like getting hit in the face with a soccer ball while watching a baseball game. I didn't expect such a blunt statement from an acquaintance, and the words smarted. *Twenty-four and no children.* I couldn't deny it, but he seemed to assume that I was childless by choice. Part of me wanted to explain that I wanted children, but I couldn't just call them down from heaven.

Instead, I said, "That's right."

Mom stepped in to reclaim the conversation. Again, I stood all but silent as they wrapped up their conversation and we left.

"Did I seem weird?" I asked. "Did I respond okay?"

Mom didn't need to ask what I meant. "You did fine." Then to reassure me, she added, "He meant it as a compliment. So many young people get married and become parents so early in life. He thinks that's unwise. He thought you felt the same as he did."

I don't think it's a bad thing to wait to start expanding your family. Timing is such a personal decision. No one should feel pressured to become parents before they feel ready. In that respect, I did not disagree with him. However, his question assumed too much for how little he knew about me.

I want children; I had wanted them for years by the time I turned twenty-four. It hurt to think that some people thought I didn't want children—even if they just thought I didn't want them yet. More than that, I felt ashamed of his praise—praise given in error. How could he know any of it? I wished he had never said anything about it. What right did he have to ask? What right did he have to either congratulate or censure me?

The words left me feeling weighted down, and I felt like I had done nothing to deserve the burden. When I was young, mother and father taught me one of weightiest words I ever learned: consequences. Our actions have consequences, they explained. Mom and Dad never issued punishments or rewards in our home. We received consequences, either good or bad. Disobedience meant bad consequences. Obedience meant good consequences.

Over the years, I've learned more about that word. I've learned that consequences can come from the decision not to act, that our actions or inactions can have effects that are un-intended, and that we can receive bad consequences when we haven't done anything wrong. It was not, is not, and never will be my duty to divulge information about when, where, or how my children come to me. Still, with people not knowing, I kept getting questions.

I know I'm not the only one, either. I have friends who have been asked if they dislike children. Others receive censure for putting career before family. Others face accusations that they must lack the proper faith or hope to conceive. Many feel their trial trivialized when others recommend "relaxing." So many people get the unwanted questions and advice. What's more, so often the person speaking has no idea what kind of barbs they are sending out. Others spew out vitriol on purpose to wound, but even they sometimes don't understand they are flinging their words at victims of fate, not choice. Words, words, words.

Trent and I both wanted to avoid talking much about the subject. However, it became evident that we would need to tell the rest of our extended families. Both of our families are close-knit. We still keep in contact with great aunts and uncles. We've gone on road trips with Trent's brother's wife's parents and sister. When my sister's husband's brother got married, we were at the reception. We still go to dinners with the happy couple.

As such, the network of people we love and who love us extends far and wide. Our loved ones feel invested in our happiness. In the early days of treatment, we hoped to be able to announce our troubles concurrent to an announcement that all our troubles were over:

"The reason we took so long to get pregnant is because we were having fertility issues, but that's okay, because we're having a baby."

It would have been so easy. The announcement of joy would have outshone the announcement of struggle. We would never need to talk about it again, we thought. But years passed, rather than months, and since the fertility treatment took so much thought and effort in our lives, every conversation seemed to hold a glimpse into our struggle. Speaking became a labyrinth to navigate: turn this way, not that. Holding the words in began to isolate us. We went from feeling like we didn't want to talk about it to feeling like we could not talk about it. The self-imposed ban rankled. And even though we wanted some release, it took time to be able to open up.

So much about infertility is so personal. The treatments, testing, and everything involve the most basic elements of what makes you up as a person. The hormones and body parts that make up your gender can be found to be lacking, too small, malfunctioning, nonexistent, or diseased. The tests involve retrieving bodily fluids. Fingers, instruments, and even needles get shoved in intimate places. There are moments when women feel their femininity ripped away, and men feel their masculinity run out of their clutching fingers. For all of us suffering infertility, there is some moment where the fact that you cannot produce children stares you in the face and makes you feel like you are missing an essential part of yourself. It is so hard to then turn to your neighbor and give them all the information that made you feel unworthy to the depths of your identity.

When we decided that we needed to release the information to our network of friends and family, we came to realize we had a whole host of decisions to make: who to extend the information to, and how much to tell. Should we reveal different amounts to different people? What should we keep private and not reveal to anyone? Information that embarrasses me might not embarrass Trent, and vice versa. After making those decisions, we sent out a brief email to those closest to us, giving a brief explanation of what was happening, why our revelation came at such a late stage in the process, and that we now felt we needed their love and support in this matter.

In other words, we needed words. They responded. There were still questions that we could not answer, but we made the decision that we would not be angry about the questions, nor would we play the evasion game.

Instead, we explained, "That's something we keep private."

In some ways, we were eager to break the silence. Still, we experienced difficulties while getting used to our newfound openness. My first instinct was to evade, and I would often need to pause before answering questions. It took effort to remember that I could talk about it, and then more effort to review what I could and could not say. I still need to sort out how much a person is likely to want to know.

It's like relearning conversation. I still get it wrong sometimes. People ask me if we have children yet, and I start to tell them my story. Then I notice the way their eyes wander—not quite able to look me in the eye—and I change the subject. Sometimes, I find I just don't have the emotional momentum to say anything more about the matter, and I can see that the person I am talking to wants nothing more than to help me unburden myself. I start to feel ashamed by the fact that I am hurting them by my silence, and I try to bolster myself to be more open—not just for me, but for them as well. Other times, I get it right.

My dad and I were video chatting one day. I explained that our doctor wanted to try to get Trent and me into optimal physical condition for in vitro, and so he prescribed some new medicines. Grinning, my dad advised me to eat more broccoli in the name of fertility. Now, by this time, I had been told to eat a myriad of strange foods to help restore fertility: frozen pineapple, high-fat dairy (I liked this idea, if truth be told), poultry products, breakfast cereals, and on and on. Dad chose broccoli because of its general healthy-ness.

In a fit of desperate hilarity, I told him everything about the different pieces of advice I'd received about fertility eating. Then, fueled by Dad's laughter and incredulity, I told him more helpful tidbits of fertile living advice. We agreed that the idea to go on an extended vacation seemed useless but desirable nonetheless. When I told him I'd heard of using egg whites for lubricant, he laughed so hard he cried. Then he called to Mom and asked if she could put a dozen eggs by the bed. Laughing too, she said no. It was a relief to just laugh about the whole situation.

Another time, I was considering a gym membership at a place near my home. The gym offered babysitting for a visit-by-visit approach or in a membership package. I skipped over that part, because I knew I wouldn't need it, but the employee giving me the tour brought it up.

"Do you have any kids yet?" he asked.

"Nope," I said.

He didn't need to know anything more. I didn't need to tell him. I didn't want to. I didn't see any reason the conversation should continue. It did.

"You planning on having them soon?"

"I don't know," I said, anxious to get on with the tour and getting a little annoyed at his persistence.

"Well, are you thinking about having one within the next year or two?"

Here is the thing. Not all infertility conversations need to be pleasant to be successful. The employee had no idea he was bringing up a tender topic. He just wanted to upsell me to a more expensive membership package. However, his actions still caused me pain. I couldn't leave him in ignorance. He might, in that ignorance, hurt someone else. To say my motivation came solely from altruistic motives, and not my own annoyance, would stretch the truth to deformity. My own frustration influenced my actions, no doubt. Still, I knew I should stop this from happening again. So, I played the TMI card. Looking hard into his eyes, I squared my shoulders.

"I don't know if I can have any kids. Ever."

It was like I had struck him. He started a bit and licked his lips.

"Oh," he said, "I'll stop talking about that, then."

I didn't get the gym membership, but I hope I did keep someone else from a high-intensity fertility question-and-answer session.

Of course, the best successful infertility conversations happen when, without my prompting at all, the other person handles everything just right. On Mother's Day, Trent and I were visiting with his sister and her family. Both sides of our family practice the same religion and attend services every Sunday. We accompanied her and her family to the chapel not too far from their home. The entire meeting focused, of course, on mothers and motherhood. I tried to stay positive by reminding myself that mothers deserve to be recognized. They need the pep talk. I myself looked forward to the day when I would sit through this type of meeting with a baby bouncing on my knee. No one set out to make me feel bad for not having children yet. At the end of the meeting, the minister asked all the mothers in the audience to stand and receive a small gift.

All the mothers began to stand as children produced little boxes of chocolates. Now, chocolates don't matter. Recognition shouldn't matter either. All I know is I wanted so badly so to be one of them. I wanted to be a mother. If everything had gone according to plan, I would be one of them. Suddenly, I felt a hand under my arm. It was my sister-in-law pulling me to my feet.

"Come on," she said. "You are standing with me."

And so I stood, arm-in-arm with my sister-in-law. It didn't change my situation at all. In fact, the Mother's Day after that, I still had no children, but I knew my sister-in-law loved me and supported me in my trial.

I remember another exchange of words that blindsided me with its sweetness. Trent and I teach a primary school class at our church. It is basically a Bible study for six-year-olds. We decided early on to add a short snack time to the schedule. During snack time, the kids can talk and run around to let off some steam. Every now and again, the children will ask us how many kids we have. We tell them we have none. Often they express their surprise; then they go back to eating.

It never hurts to answer their questions. They're six years old. In their experience, married adults who like children are parents, or soon will be. They don't think anything of it; they don't judge us. In fact, they often forget they've already asked us, and ask again. On one occasion, I sat next to two of the little girls. When one asked if we had kids, I said no, but that we looked forward to becoming parents one day. I thought that was the end of it. But then the second little girl gave me a penetrating look. Whatever she saw in my face, I don't know. All I know is what she said.

"My aunt and uncle adopted their kids," she said, her sweet face full of sympathy.

I couldn't believe she saw the connection.

"I bet they love their kids very much," I said.

"Yes," she said. "Just as much as my parents love me."

I am not just a consumer of words. I am a producer of words—most of the time. Sometimes, I am stunned to silence.

Answers

Yes, we've been married for long enough,
And yes, we've been trying for long enough.
Yes, I like, even love children,
And, yes, I want them.
Yes, we've read the Bible,
And yes, we know it is our duty to be parents.
Yes, we've prayed about it,
And we are still waiting to know why this is happening.
Yes, our parents certainly want grandchildren,
And they are sharing our grief, I'm sure.
No, we aren't afraid of having children,
But we are afraid of why we don't have them.
No, we aren't delaying,
But treatments, paperwork, and healing take so much time.
No, we aren't ashamed we have no children,
But the medical reasons sometimes feel humiliating.
No, it's not a sin for you to be curious,
But if I'd wanted your confidence, I'd have sought it.
No, I don't mind your asking,
But I do.

Full Disclosure

*I*f I'm willing to talk about a subject, I give information out like penny-store candy. If I'm the least bit reluctant, I can clamp down like a mollusk. For example, I've never been the type of person who likes to talk about my body. I figure that my body is nobody's business but my own. Which, of course, drives my doctors mad.

My least favorite bodily discussions are feminine issues and sex. I don't like having to answer detailed questions about my menstrual cycle. I don't like pelvic exams or pap smears. I don't like it when the doctors check my ovaries or take measurements of my uterus. Even before fertility treatments, I didn't like doctors' appointments.

I'm not quite sure where my reluctance started. I did grow up in a conservative, religious home, which might lead some to believe my reluctance stems from a closed-mouth attitude at home. But unlike some religious households, we were very open about sexuality. When I was eight years old, my parents gave me "the talk." After sending the younger children off to bed, they asked me to sit on the couch. Taking chairs from the dining room, they sat across from me. My parents then gave a detailed, but not graphic, explanation about puberty, love, and sex. At the time, the information overwhelmed me.

As the talk wound to a close, my parents said, "We want you to know that you can ask us any questions you want. You never need to feel embarrassed, okay? You'll probably hear people talking about it at school, especially as you get older. If anything sounds confusing to you, just come and talk to us, okay?"

I sat there feeling flabbergasted, but I nodded.

"Do you have any questions about what we just said?"

Yes.

"No, thank you."

Mom and Dad sat and waited for a moment. They weren't menacing, just waiting. When I still didn't budge, they sat back. Neither looked the least bit uncomfortable.

"If you think of anything later, you can ask. Alright?"

"Okay."

I did get up the courage to ask them questions. In fact, I felt more comfortable asking my parents about sex or bodily changes than I ever did asking my doctor. And I absolutely trusted them to answer my questions more than my teachers. I still remember, in middle school, when we began taking the "puberty classes." After watching an uncomfortable video of bad acting and even worse euphemisms, the teachers asked for questions. I didn't ask any. I'd already talked to my parents about everything covered in the video. None of my peers asked anything either. In fact, they shifted in discomfort, refusing to look anyone in the face. The teachers, seeing the reluctance of some of my peers, insisted we all write at least one question on a piece of paper before they allowed us to leave class. Their insistence infuriated me. I liked my teachers, and I trusted them. Still, I did not want to ask them questions about puberty. So, as my only means of showing my displeasure, I wrote a snarky question:

"If chocolate isn't supposed to cause zits, why do I get zits every time I eat chocolate?"

I didn't get an answer.

When I got older, my periods turned from an annoyance to an outright hardship. The pain become so unmanageable, I sought treatment. During that first appointment, I got a taste of how thorough doctors' questions could get. I think I must have been fourteen at the time. Though already at my adult height, my colt-ish clumsiness showed that my soul still felt three inches shorter than my actual height. Despite my clumsiness, I often garnered some confidence from my new ability to set my feet flat on the floor while sitting in a chair. However, the exam table left my elongated legs dangling, thwarting even this small comfort. At my invitation, Mom joined me in the examination room, though she sat in the chair.

After a short greeting, the doctor began.

"Are your periods regular?"

Easy enough to answer.

"Yes."

"How long do they last?"

"Five to seven days."

Isn't that the norm?

"Are they heavy or light?"

Ew.

"Um . . . heavy."

"Are they painful?"

Holy cow, yes.

"Yes."

"How painful?"

Painful enough for me to be willing to talk to you. Can I say the word "hellish"?

"Hellish."

"Do you experience any clots?"

I don't think I can do this.

"Uh . . ."

"And is the blood red or brown?"

I didn't want them to know. I don't want them to know. It's gross. It's bloody and gross and I'd rather not say, thank you very much. But that isn't the type of answer a doctor likes to hear. It's also not the type of answer that can get you any help. I must wrestle with myself to answer.

As the questions get more detailed, my answers take longer to come. My husband, who has started to accompany me to every doctor visit per my request, gives me encouraging looks as I try to think of a way to answer the doctor's questions and not die of shame. When infertility treatment started, the questions got more personal.

"How often do you have sex?"

I don't want to tell them how often my husband and I are intimate. That's an intimate question. But I want to have a baby, so I tell them how often we have sex.

"Do you have hair under your arms and in the genital area?"

That one is easy, because, really I don't care if they know that I need to shave my armpits. Most women do. As for the other hair, after the required exams would take place, the doctor and I would have no secrets anyway.

"Do you grow any hair on your stomach, inner thighs, face, or breasts? If so, is it dark or light? Coarse or fine?"

Now that is something I definitely don't want to talk about: unusual hair. It makes me wonder if they ever ask women if they have cellulite, and if so where? And how deep are the dimples? But again, I want a child with every inch of my imperfect body. The question about hair is significant. If there is hair that grows in unusual places for a woman, that is a warning sign of polycystic ovarian syndrome (PCOS), a genetic, but treatable, endocrine disorder that can cause or contribute to infertility. I know that it serves a purpose to answer, and so I do, in a long string of monosyllables.

"How is your libido?"

I just told you how often we have sex. Guess.

"Oh. Uh. Well . . . fine. It's . . . uh . . . fine."

"Are your periods regular?"

The questions are as cyclical as the menstrual cycle they are asking about. Every new doctor needs to ask. I tell myself that they don't ask in order to be nosy. They don't ask for the pleasure of making me squirm. I know all these things. There's just an emotional disconnect. I know that these doctors and nurses are trying to help me in my goal. I'm only hindering them if I try to withhold information. I just make it harder on myself when I try to hold on to every scrap of data I don't need to expound upon. Really, it might turn out to be relevant.

There are so many different prices to pay for a child. One of them is full disclosure. I have spent my time dolling out facts, paying to give them to doctors who have paid to learn to decode the complex clues given by a body. At the beginning of this ordeal, I decided that I would give the world to have a child. It was an easy thing to say because I have no world to give. I don't own a single scrap of the world. Even the place where I live is borrowed.

Instead, I am paying with the only thing I somewhat own: myself. I go to the doctor to participate in a confession of the inadvertent sins of the body. With each detailed imperfection, I hope that I can be shriven, absolved, and produce a child. Trent attends the same confession, and I don't even know what it costs him to answer those questions. I know what it costs me to see him struggle to answer them. I wonder if it costs as much for him to see me struggle to answer.

I don't even know if we can be saved. The more information we give, the more medical absolution we seem to stand in need of. While religion can offer forgiveness and rebirth from almost any sin, the sciences of this life cannot offer a surety of a first birth.

Full disclosure is a currency towards a vaporous dream. Every embarrassing admission gets me closer to a golden maybe.

The real reward for my own full disclosure is the answers that come from the doctor. He, too, is bound to dole out information. The more I give him, the more he can give me. After the poking and prodding, the blood tests, and the pelvic exams, I get to ask the doctor what it all means.

"How did my cervical mucus look?"

"Should it be thicker or not as thick?"

"How do my progesterone levels look?"

"If I took more vitamins, would it help our fertility situation?"

"What are the odds of [insert treatment here] working?"

"How long should we wait?"

"How much will that cost?"

"When will we know?"

"Are you sure?"

I get the answers from the doctor, and I get the hope toward the maybe. I think about the fact that I get what I trade for, that I now know more, and so does the doctor. I think about the lack of certainty. I think about how I want this trade of information to be worth it. I have chosen to look more into why I can't have children. The blame is mine, not the doctor's.

I want to be stoic about the information I give. After all, if I want any chance to get successful treatment, the doctors need information. I keep hoping that I can stop answering questions and start getting the results instead. I keep wondering when I'll be saved, when I'll get the payout for my investment, or however you want to explain it. What I want is a baby. I want it all to be worth it. I want to look into my child's eyes and say to myself, "I sacrificed my privacy and my comfort, and it doesn't even matter now, because it's worth it. This child is worth it. "

I have another doctor's appointment to go to with my husband this week. In the spirit of full disclosure, I know there's no way to be sure this will get me the result I want. It bothers me that I don't have that assurance. I'm going to tell them everything I can anyway.

Maybe

"Maybe" has a bitter, lasting taste to it,
almost like algae on the tongue
or sand in the teeth.
Bacterial-flavored slime that won't slip past the tongue,
or desert-tasting grit that won't un-grip the teeth.

It's not so blunt as "No,"
which is more like a short, hard flick
to the uvula.
"No" has often left me gagging, gasping:
airless and rebellious.
With "Maybe," I spend all my energy on trying to
    somehow swallow.
I can't rebel, can't gag, can't spit.
But at least I can breathe.

Creation

I am not one of those that create,
though I know the methods
of the laudable creators.

With his own hands, immortal God
molded man from the dust
and carved woman from a rib,
both in a single day's time.

In the protection of their own wombs,
mortal women craft children
over a longer span of nine months.

And, oh, if only I could reach out my hands
and mold the dust into a little living man,
or carve a rib into a little living woman,
or hold a child in my womb;
by whatever means God would grant me,
with whatever time God would award me,
I simply long to create.

PART EIGHT

TO FRIENDS
AND FAMILY

What to Say

I can see it in your eyes when you ask me—that swift spasm in the iris, the sudden dilation of the pupil. Then the thoughts run across the whites of your eyes as if they're being handwritten. I can see that you worry. You worry that now is not a good time to ask, that you will say the wrong thing, that you will trivialize our problems or that you will overemphasize our problems, that we have been silent because the news is bad and we don't want to share it, that you are asking too many questions or not enough. You worry I'll feel pressured to answer. You worry that you shouldn't have brought it up.

I worry that you will get so worried about saying the right thing that you won't say anything at all.

I know what it feels like to be on the outside of a tragedy. I remember facing friends who suffered a great loss or disappointment and not knowing what to say or give. I wanted to be their beacon of hope, their consolation, their healing balm. All I could really think of was how woefully inadequate I was to fill the space left by their loss and disappointed hopes. Now, being the one suffering disappointment, I often feel at a loss to explain what it is I need. Because I don't know either. To tell the truth, I sometimes get distracted by what is gone and cannot be replaced. So, I sit there, looking into your eyes thinking, *I wish I could help you help me.*

I'm sure you've noticed that, for the most part, I've just been muddling through this. Through all the muddle and muck, I know there have been some awkward moments, hurt feelings, and times of loneliness. Even so, there have been no lost friendships and no irreparable damage done. That being acknowledged, I think it means both of us did a few things right. I'm still learning what to do, and I'm sure you are, too. Still, I feel like we've reached a point where the moments of awkwardness aren't so frequent. So, I decided to write down a few things about the confusing trek in the hope that it will help you understand the past, help us in future conversation, and maybe help someone else navigate this quagmire.

Trent and I took more than a year to start telling people about our infertility struggle. In fact, we did a sort of slow release, starting with family and close friends. Then we told more friends. Now we tell anyone who asks. We didn't plan on this time-released method of revelation. In fact, for a long time, we just figured we wouldn't ever need to tell most people. We assumed that the infertility would come and go. Life would continue on in a normal fashion, and the amount of time it took to get pregnant would prove irrelevant.

We didn't want to overreact. We thought an early announcement of our troubles would be the equivalent of telling everyone we might have skin cancer after getting a bad sunburn at the beach. It's possible to get skin cancer from a bad burn, but in all likelihood, we'd just be uncomfortable for a few days and the sunburn would only serve as a learning experience. Jumping the gun like that would only make people upset and worried, and in the end, we'd need to take time and energy to tell everyone that we're just fine.

After we were sure that our infertility would be a continuing problem, we expanded the realm of people we told. Even then, we waited to tell most of our friends. The truth is, telling people about the hardest thing that has ever happened in your life takes effort. It's like confronting the situation all over again. Our reserves of energy needed to be divided between normal life, seeking treatment, and informing our family of our progress. The division of energy caused our reserves to run low. Most times, our choices of whom to tell, when to tell them, and how much to tell were influenced more by our own energy levels than by how much we loved or trusted the person involved. After the slow release, we had a vast network of wonderful people to support us, including you. It's quite possible that I don't even remember when I told you anything. What I do remember is that the initial responses from our friends and family helped so much. We felt loved and enveloped in a safe sphere. And we were exhausted.

It's been difficult establishing this network of support. It's exhausting, but the hardest part is figuring out how on earth the support group will function and how we can spare you unneeded pain. Believe it or not, the support group is not just there for us. All of you are our family and our friends, and even though the news affects us most directly, it affects all of you, too.

My parents and parents-in-law are devastated. Their main

concern is for our welfare, but they, too, are disappointed and upset. They are missing their grandchildren. Our siblings are missing their nieces and nephews. Our nieces and nephews are missing their cousins. Our friends feel such sympathy (and sometimes empathy) for us.

To my family, I am heartbroken for you who are missing out on your grandchildren, your nieces and nephews, your cousins. To my friends, thank you for your sympathy (and I'm so sorry if you can empathize). I try to keep your heartbreak in mind when I talk to you. I try to remember the fact that you are invested in this, too. That having company on this journey means I'm obliged to share the pain, because how can you come with me if I leave you behind?

After we issued the invitation to join our support group, after we felt the relief of your company, and after the exhaustion of all that work, our journey began in earnest. But the strangest thing is that ordinary life kept happening right alongside it. You have your own priorities that need attention; Trent and I have other goals we work toward. And as real, imperfect life continues, real and imperfect things are said. I remember so many conversations with so many different people in my support group.

I remember one day, I was so tired. Trent and I hadn't made any progress in our fertility situation. Something else was wrong, too. I can't even remember what it was—maybe I was sick or Trent was in the middle of a stressful dental course. Whatever it was, I was drained, and it was that moment when you asked about infertility. I bet you were worried that this alignment of circumstances might come about. And you must have worried if, by asking at a difficult time, you would hurt me or make my pain worse. I wonder if you worried it would make me angry? You probably noticed the way my face grew tight, and then you saw the pain. The thing is, you didn't cause me that pain. It's alright to ask me from time to time how things are going. If you do, there will be times when you ask at a bad time. That isn't your fault, and I know it. You should never feel bad for being concerned for my welfare. That being said, if I change the subject, wait a while to bring it up again.

Another day, you asked me a question; I can't even remember what it was. I answered, but I changed the subject quickly. I hope you know it was because I was enjoying your company. I was so glad to be having a moment of normalcy with you. Sometimes, it just feels nice to remember that there is a life beyond this trial—that happiness can come from more than one source. I didn't change the subject because of a lack of trust. I changed it because I value my time with you.

That time you asked me something and I told you I don't share that information, it wasn't because I'd suddenly decided I didn't want your confidence. It was because it was something that embarrasses either Trent or me. And we've agreed never to talk about it outside the home. It's not that we can't stand you knowing. It's that we can't stand *anyone* knowing. Sometimes we are just so embarrassed by what is happening we can't bear to put our shame to words. I feel like, in order to achieve our goals, I must tell our doctors everything, to let the doctor look at everything. And I hate that necessity. While I know that you love me and would never look at me with disdain, sometimes I don't want to give anyone that opportunity, even knowing you would never take it—possibly because whatever it is I am not sharing makes me look at myself differently.

Then, a few days later, you were shocked by what I was willing to share. I could see the shock in the way you couldn't stop looking at me. Thank you for explaining to me that you were shocked by my openness, not by what I shared. There is a confident part of myself that knows you will love me no matter what. There is also a frightened and vulnerable part that needs to hear you say it.

I also wanted you to know that I received the invitation to your baby shower. It must have been difficult for you to decide whether or not to send it—wondering whether I would take offense or if I would feel jealous or if it would simply make me hurt. I'll tell you what I told my younger sister one day. I knew that she and her husband might be trying for children soon, so I took her aside and let her know that if she got pregnant, I wanted to be among the first people she told.

"I'm already missing out on happy news for me; I don't want to miss out on your happy news."

That being said, I did cry when, a few months later, she let me know that she was expecting. I cried both because I was happy for her and sad for me. The tears were a price I knew I would pay, and I have never regretted paying that price. I might have cried when I got your invitation, too. I can't remember for sure, because some days are different. And because some days are different, I might or might not come to the baby shower. It's not that I am not happy for you. It's not that I'm offended or jealous or angry. I just want you to enjoy your day, and I know that my breaking down in tears as you open presents wouldn't add to your happiness or mine. Expect a card and present in the mail.

You might also remember a few times, early on in this trial, when I seemed to give mixed signals. How one day, I said, "I need some space." Then, the next day, I called to talk to you and told you I felt lonely. Or the time I said, "I just feel like I need some distraction," and then the next day, I turned down an opportunity to go to a play because I felt "too overwhelmed." My only excuse is I've never done this before. I never expected this trial, so I often don't know what I need, much less how to communicate those needs. I know my inconsistencies and confusion cause grief. I know because I see that grief in my friends, in my husband, and in myself. The best advice I can give for this situation is to just be there in general. If I ask for space, don't always insist on being with me, but do call from time to time. If I say I need distraction, let me know about things I might be interested in, but don't get offended if I decline. I'm just as confused as you are.

I'm sure you know by now that some people know less than you do or maybe some know more. There have been times when I've left out long swaths of the story and then suddenly called to tell you amazing or terrible news. There are days when I'm so down that you worry if I will be okay. There are days when I am so hopeful it's both encouraging and heartbreaking. You've heard me hiss out bitter and angry things; you've heard me give magnanimous declarations. You have seen me struggle through this, and no doubt about it, it has been a struggle. And despite it all, you're still talking to me.

I know you still wonder what to say to me. The best advice I can give for now is this: say something. I love talking to you.

What Not to Say

*N*ow comes the uncomfortable moment when I acknowledge that sometimes people say things that light my brain on fire with sadness, discomfort, and even anger. Most of the time, I don't address the situation. I just want to leave, extinguish my flaming brain, and take a nap. Other times, the scorching of my synapses lets loose a whole other side of me where I do address the situation, but not in a way that will really help any of us. Here, in this brief moment, I want to address some of the most common things people say that can (perhaps unintentionally) cause sizzled synapsis, hurt feelings, and general distress. I want to confront the situation before my emotions get affected by that mental fire. I want to say just enough without keeping silent or getting angry. And so, in this list, I will explain what it is that hurts, why it hurts me, and what I would prefer you say or do.

Why?

This is the word that most often seems to pop up in infertility conversations.

"*Why* don't you have children yet?"

"*Why* do you spend so much money on fertility treatments?"

And it pops up so often because human beings always ask "why" when our expectations are shaken. For example, in the normal goings-on of everyday life, couples like Trent and me (married, young, in love, and fond of children) have children fairly soon after getting married. Most of our family, friends, and acquaintances expected us to be expecting within a few short months of our wedding vows. So, when years passed and we still had no children, people began to ask, "Why?" Now, the reason the word *why* hurts so much is because many of the answers are painful and private.

"We don't have children because we are infertile, meaning that our lifelong dream of becoming parents might never be realized."

"We spend so much money on fertility treatments because the only other alternative was to give up our entire life plan."

I don't necessarily want to say these things. I might decide to confide in you, but I feel like the question, "Why?" backs me into a corner—especially when the question has to do with decisions Trent and I have made regarding our treatment for infertility.

"*Why* in vitro and not adoption?"

"*Why* did you go to that clinic and not this one?"

These questions threaten to go even deeper into the realms of what a couple might not feel comfortable talking about. The route to each person's path to parenthood is highly personalized—each choice is motivated by each person's opportunities, finances, moral beliefs, and even health.

The problem with *why* is that it leaves so little wiggle room. The word traps me. I feel like I can't choose how much I want to explain. There's so much that went into why, and so much of it is something I choose to hold close, not to share. The best questions allow me the freedom to give as much or as little information as possible.

For example, instead of asking, "Why don't you have children yet?" you could ask, "Any exciting plans in the future?" Because, yes, I do have exciting plans. I might not tell you about whether or not we are planning on pursuing fertility treatments, but you will hear more about what is going on in our lives.

Instead of asking, "Why in vitro and not adoption?" you could ask, "How did you decide what you wanted to do?" Then I can feel free to tell you only about the moments that made me cry with excitement and leave out the times when I felt as insecure as quicksand. Sometimes I am not strong enough to relive those quicksand moments. These open questions help me to open up.

Using *why* inappropriately isn't the worst infertility faux pas that someone can make when asking questions. We who suffer infertility can usually see that there was no intent to offend with *why*. There are other questions that cause us much more discomfort.

Questions That Reveal Assumptions

I've been lucky. I haven't gotten many of these. However, I know many people who have had to face them. The questions usually go something like this:

"Did you ever think that maybe you aren't supposed to have children?"

The thinly veiled assumption here is twofold. The first assumption is that those who suffer infertility should probably live childless. Infertility is not the sentence of childlessness that it used to be, just as cancer is no longer the death sentence it once was. Infertility is a treatable disease with many causes.

The other assumption is that the couple hasn't considered living childless. When you are struck with infertility, you have to make choices: Do you seek treatment? Do you adopt? Do you live childless? And let me say from personal experience, it's a wrenching time when you sit across from your spouse and consider the rest of your life. Each path has its own emotional and physical costs.

Others assumption-ridden questions include:

"Don't you like children?"

This one assumes that I am childless because I don't want children, and that cuts me to the core. The desire for children makes up such a great portion of who I am. When people assume that I chose to have no children, I feel a pang deep inside my empty womb. When people go a step further and assume I simply don't like children, I feel more than misunderstood. I feel mislabeled, misconstrued, missed. They missed one of the most important parts of who I am.

"Have you thought about having children yet?"

Yes, actually. Sometimes it's all I think about. And I don't like the assumption that I might not have.

"Whose fault is it?"

When people ask me this one, I cringe. First of all, it implies that one of us is "at fault," when neither of us did anything that would have caused our infertility. Infertility, in general, comes about because of bodily problems that you were born with or developed in adolescence. Sometimes, it comes about because of abuse or injury. No matter the reason, very few cases come from active self sabotage. The connotation that blame can be assigned to the victim of infertility only hurts the victim.

That being said, it is okay to ask, "Have the doctors figured out what's wrong?" That question carries no assumptions. And those questions are the best ones to ask. Not all infertility faux pas have to do with questions, though. Different types of commentary also cause stress.

Repetitive and/or Unsolicited Advice

I'm not sure there is any couple suffering infertility that hasn't been through these. They usually begin with, "Have you tried…?" and can end with anything in the range from "diet change" to "deep tissue massage" to "research groups" to "medicinal teas."

During the early stages of an advice-giving conversation, I don't really feel that uncomfortable. In fact, if I haven't heard of it, and it seems like something that might work for me, I will ask for more information. No, it's only when the advice persists that I start to get upset. Once I say I'm not interested, I don't want to continue the conversation. Some do continue, and I find there are usually two reasons they persist.

"My sister/friend/neighbor tried it, and it worked."

If that is so, I'm very glad, but fertility treatment is highly individualized. I have decided against treatment options for many different reasons. The treatment might not address the fertility issues Trent and I face, or it might be too expensive, too risky, or too uncomfortable. We might not get along well with the doctor that offers that treatment or might want to stay with the doctor we already have. We might find the treatment doesn't match our moral ideals. Though we haven't reached this point yet, we might one day decide that we need to stop fertility treatments altogether. Whatever the reason, it should be enough for me to say, "No, thank you."

The other reason people persist is that they think, *I can help you.* Which makes it that much harder to tell them no. I do need help. I know it, but I need to be the one to communicate my needs. If I say, "No," I have a reason for doing so.

There is, however, one piece of unsolicited advice that I think should never be given. I'm speaking of the ever-nerve-grating, "Just relax and let it happen."

Relaxation can help with infertility treatments, yes. However, the causes of infertility should not be glossed over and they need to be addressed. Sometimes, the treatment of infertility can help doctors discover bodily defects, the treatment of which can bring about a general increase in health. Sometimes the causes of infertility can be dangerous illnesses, including cancer. Other times, when no defect is found, the seeking of treatment can at least erase the feelings of guilt caused by inaction.

Those of us who suffer infertility need to relax because the situation is stressful. But we do not need to be told to relax. Instead, what we need is a friend with whom we can relax.

The Story

I have heard this story often. And it is always meant to comfort. The first few times I heard The Story, it did offer comfort. Now, it only makes me sad, because it cannot and will not happen for us. It's impossible. Truly impossible. The Story is usually told when I reveal that I am seeking treatment for infertility, often when I am talking about in vitro. Every story varies slightly in its composition, as do the characters, but the core is always the same:

"I knew a couple who tried for children for years and then, right after they had a child (through expensive treatment or adoption), they got pregnant."

I am beginning to suspect that everyone knows the exact same couple. Now, I do like success stories, and I recognize this is one of them. However, the success story that will help me is the one that most resembles what might happen for me. While going through in vitro, I want to hear stories of couples who conceived through that process, even if it wasn't on the first attempt. When going through adoption, I want to hear stories of adoptions where the birth family and the adoptive family both felt good about the adoption process. Help me to know good things can come from the road I'm taking.

The Biological Clock

I already know it's there. I know the weeks are building to months and the months are building into years. I know, and that fact looms below me like a great white shark. Even with the quick action my husband and I took to fight infertility, age might just catch us in its jaws. That clock clicks a relentless, sinister rhythm in my head, and when you tell me about it, you are only composing lyrics on top of that constant, frightening metronome.

"Are you pregnant?"

No, I'm not. And it's best not to ask this question to anyone, anyway.

PART NINE

COPING

Not Today

I 'm not going to think about it today. I refuse. Which, of course, means I can't go to the supermarket. They carry clothes at the supermarket, and not just adult clothes, but children's clothes, and not just children's clothes, but baby's clothes. I can't look at baby's clothes today. So, I won't go to the supermarket.

I could go to the mall. But then, the supermarket problem is compounded. There are entire stores dedicated to babies and kids and even expectant mothers. I can't go there, to the land of toy stores and teenagers. Babies grow up to be teenagers, too. I am not old enough to be the mother of teenage children. But I worry that by the time I have teen children, I'll be the age of their peer's grandparents. The mall is out of the question.

I also can't go out to the restaurant. Whenever I sit at a restaurant table, I'm seated near children. It must be fate. Well-behaved kids make me yearn for parenthood. I glance over to see the happy family being polite to the waitress and the three little kids coloring on the paper menus they were given, the mom and dad looking like they are my age. Misbehaving ones bring on a sort of sadistic self-pity. *At least you don't have to deal with that. Wouldn't it be great if you had to deal with that?* No. I can't go to a restaurant.

I can't go for a walk, either. I'm too near a park. The kids are laughing, and I can see the moms all talking together on the benches that line the playground like guard posts. I could go and talk to the moms. I know a few of them; some are even good friends, but on days like today, I worry I'll be jealous. I don't want to be jealous. I don't even want to think about how it's real. Depending on which way I leave the house, I can avoid seeing them, but I don't want to risk hearing. So, a walk is out. Maybe I shouldn't go out today.

Still, I can't just sit and do nothing. That won't help. An idle mind has a horrible habit of wrenching up bad thoughts. I think a mind wants stimulation, and what is more stimulating than sad thoughts? The dishes always need doing and the carpet could always use another vacuum and maybe I could do some ironing. Of course, these things leave my mind to wander. So, maybe I can watch the TV while I work.

But no. I can't watch TV. There are all those commercials with moms choosing peanut butter brands and otherwise providing their families with the world's most superb products. The tissue commercials make me sniffle; those ones with moms wiping noses that are supposed to be snotty, but look amazingly clean. Card commercials make me wish for a tissue myself, with moms giving kids cards for graduating, participating in sports, Christmas. I can't take it. No good. No TV.

An audio book. I like audio books. They can keep my mind busy enough. I'll listen to a childhood favorite. Except, no. That one makes me think about how I want to read it to my kids someday. Not that one. The romance novel? No. Just, no. The one about the orphan? No. Okay, none of that.

Well, reading will be off the list, too. I could write, except that most of what I write has been about infertility the past few months. My mind pulls the infertility essays to my typing fingers like cotton candy to a child's mouth. Maybe I could just write a poem about something beautiful: a nice autumn scene painted out in words. Like the times when I would jump in giant piles of leaves at the park with my family because only sagebrush grew near our house. And, oh, how I want to live in a place where my children will know both the smell of sagebrush and the scent leaves. I'm done with that poem idea. I'll move on.

Maybe I'll just surf on the internet. Of course, I might see another pregnancy announcement on social media again. I don't want to fight that battle between happiness for my friend and sadness for me.

I could take a nap. That sounds nice. I've been a little tired today. It might be nice to just sleep for a bit. But then again, like Hamlet says, dreams aren't predictable in their content. I've been having a lot of dreams about pregnancy or adoption. In fact, the other day, I remember waking up to Trent kissing me and the first words out of my mouth were, "Would you like to adopt a little boy named Pablo?"—Pablo being the most recent child I dreamed into existence. In my present moods, I'm more than sure that I would dream up another child I will leave behind on waking.

I don't want to think about it today. I don't want to think about it today. I don't want to think about it today. But it's as if there is no person, place, or thing that can't be a stimulus toward thinking about the fact that infertility is a part of my life. I don't want to think about it. But the harder I try not to think about it, the more I can see it.

The thing is, my only certainty about infertility is that it is an ever-present part of my life. I can't "not think about it" today, because it is still true today. I map out what I want to do with my life based on my situation in relation to my infertility. I don't want to think about it today, but I still want to move forward with my life. I want to go out to the supermarket and the restaurants. I want to watch television, listen to audio books, and read. I want to be able to surf the net and take a nap. I want to be able to let my mind wander.

If what matters most is not thinking about it, I would need insulation, encapsulating myself in an alternate reality so cushioned it might just suffocate me. I don't want to think about it today, but I think I would rather be able to breathe.

Cheapskates

rent and I have always been frugal. We both came from frugal households. As the oldest child in my family, I can still remember a time when we couldn't afford cable. Trent, as the second youngest in a family of six children, grew up with the flurry of coupon cutting. Both of us remember hand-me-downs. I got the outfits of my older cousins. Trent got his hand-me-downs from his older brothers.

In our younger college careers, we both lived in old apartments, the ones where we share three bedrooms and one fridge with six people. In one of my places, there was a hole in the floor. The managers repaired it by stretching linoleum over the gap. Very economical. Every time my roommates and I stepped in it, we sank ankle-deep into the flooring. Trent's apartment boasted one bathroom. One bathroom for six men meant short showers in a very grimy tub.

When we first got married, we had approximately one thousand dollars to our name. Though each of us had secured jobs, we also attended school. I worked an internship that, with a twenty-five-cent raise, brought my wages up to $7.75 an hour. Trent joined a catering job, earning twenty-five cents less than me. We paid a little more than four hundred dollars a month in rent. I tried to keep our grocery expenses down to about forty-five dollars a week. Our date budget consisted of a meager ten dollars a week. Even with those strictures, we needed financial help from our parents.

When we started trying for children, our financial prospect looked better. At the time, I worked for a software training company as a technical writer. We'd also managed to earn substantial amounts during the previous summer. Still, we knew we would need to maintain strict economy to prepare for the expenses to come. We scrimped and saved, making sure that we could pay for labor and delivery, as well as the baby's clothes, diapers, and other needs. When we found we would need to save up for in vitro, we felt absolute shock. Not just shock at the severity of the diagnosis. Sticker shock.

Only about 3 percent of couples experiencing infertility go through with in vitro. I can't blame them. Besides the considerations of health and prognosis, the cost can be as much as a brand new car. And that is before prenatal care and labor and delivery. Plus, there's no guarantee that the in vitro would work. None. There's just a prognosis. We decided we would do it, at all costs. So, we saved.

It's not an easy thing to do, saving money while in the middle of gaining an education. My entry-level contracted technical writing position didn't yield a lot of excess income. Trent made more in scholarships than I did working, and we needed that money to pay for tuition and books and equipment fees and so forth. With so little income and so much money needed to achieve our goals, we economized as much as possible.

We don't buy a lot of things. We don't go out to eat very

much. The gifts we give are not expensive ones. We seem like cheapskates. Sometimes, I feel a deep embarrassment. I want to give wedding presents like crock pots and pancake griddles. Instead, we assemble little date-night kits of a movie and popcorn. I also wish that I could say yes to more activities with friends. Every now and again, we will splurge and go to an evening movie or out to a restaurant. We often wind up having to say no to invitations. I feel bad, because I like spending time with friends and family. It's just I want to become a parent even more.

I sometimes worry that I am offending people. I try to explain that we can't afford to go out all that often, but there are so few people who "can't afford" to go out to a movie or buy a nice wedding present. It's just so hard to tell people that the reason you can't go out is that every dollar you spend gets weighed against having a child. It sounds melodramatic, even to me. And I'm living it. Sometimes, at the supermarket, I'll stand paralyzed between a twelve dollar roast and a ten dollar packet of ground hamburger not sure which is the better deal.

Once, I went out shopping with my sister. I needed a new winter top, and she needed a new dress. After finding a nice dress, my sister held up a soft-looking gray sweater. It was on sale for twenty dollars.

"This could be cute," she said.

"For you or for me?" I asked.

"For you," she said.

"Oh, it does look very cute," I said, "but it's a little much."

Her eyebrows raised, but I tried to explain.

"Still saving for the baby," I said.

She nodded, and gave me a look of sympathy. I later found one for less than fifteen dollars. Four dollars isn't a lot, but saving four dollars here and there adds up.

The world seems to think that you can't set a price on dreams. It has the same view about friendships. Now, I don't wish to be crass, but dreams come with enormous price tags, even the dream of parenthood. There is also a price associated with having and maintaining friendships. I feel like the people I love and the dreams I dream are of infinite worth to me, and if I could, I would pay anything and everything for both. Unfortunately, I live in a world so finite that I can't afford to give anything and everything to either one. I give time, invest what money I can, and then hope my friends recognize my efforts for what they are.

I use coupons to buy everything from groceries to gifts. The gifts I give are cheesy; the restaurants we go to don't serve unprocessed cheese. I don't buy name-brand jeans or even name-brand mustard. I wash my Ziploc bags by hand. We go to the dollar movie theater and don't go to dinner beforehand. Most of my clothes are second-hand or clearance items. My wardrobe doesn't change much from summer to winter, except that, in winter, I wear more layers. Most of Trent's clothes come from his high school years. He doesn't go out for lunch when he's at school. Most of the new books we read come from the library. My husband worked himself to the bone to get a great scholarship so that we could afford dental school. In the winter, we turn the heater down to about fifty degrees at night. After dinner, we open up the oven as it cools from cooking to take full advantage of the extra heat.

To look at us and our behavior, you would think that my husband and I are cheapskates. We're not. We are extravagant. We are willing to pay all the money not spent on the necessities on one single thing: helping our family grow.

Spaces

$\mathcal{T}$ rent and I have been battling our infertility for years now. Though the struggle has been life altering and time consuming, the battles themselves come in short spurts. Intervals stretch between the times we receive clusters of test results, treatment options, and the treatments themselves. The hours have built and bunched around us, and though I can still remember that day when the doctor came in with so much bad news, we've lived hundreds of moments since then.

In the early stages of our infertility treatment, I let those gaps between results slip past without much notice. Trent and I were hyper-focused on becoming parents. We'd separated our lives out into milestones we wanted to achieve. Our sudden arrests in movement toward one goal proved damning.

I don't mean to say that we failed to accomplish anything in that time. I mean to say that our other accomplishments felt like consolation prizes. Our efforts toward parenthood dominated our attention. Even now, we spend months in between pushes forward. It seems like we make crawling progress; then we leap into a sprint.

My friends who also suffer the trial of infertility often express that same sort of pent-up frustration. It feels like time is passing, but life gets put on hold. Trent and I worry about making plans that might interfere with fertility treatments. In order to afford treatment, we must remain frugal. For every purchase above a certain amount, we weigh it against the possibility of having a child. The thought of running out of money or being out of town for a possible round of in vitro frightens us. One month's delay in infertility is never just one month's delay. It's always at least ten.

The problem is humans don't do well with stagnation. We are beings of movement. Even our own bodies show evidence of our need to progress. If we sit still for too long, our blood clots. If we keep from exercising, our bodies become susceptible to chronic diseases. Likewise, if we fail to make progress towards our goals, we sink into a hellish depression.

The dilemma Trent and I often face is this: do we abandon our goal of having children and risk being forever disappointed, or do we stay steadfast and risk stagnation? We tried to find a halfway point. It's a shifting, perilous middle ground to balance living the life we live now and looking forward to the life we want. A few years ago, we started looking into the spaces between. They were filled with so little, it was like we vanished in the times we weren't trying for children.

For me, one incident brought home how much we had let ourselves slip. After finishing a late winter dinner with my sister and her husband, Trent offered to go pull the car around and pick me up. The moment the door closed behind him, my sister Jessica, leaned toward me and said,

"Is Trent okay?"

The question took me off guard. I tried to think if Trent said or did anything negative during dinner. No specific instances came to mind.

"What do you mean?" I asked.

"He just isn't smiling as much. He hardly laughed or even talked tonight."

She was right. Without my realizing it, Trent had spent most of the evening in complete silence. The fact that this behavior failed to register in my mind made my stomach sink. Trent and I both thought we could hide our sadness, but no. Instead of fooling those closest to us, we had only fooled ourselves. It took my sister's question to make us realize that our preoccupation and grief were noticeable to others.

When we were out and about, we did try to put forth a brave front. Most of our friends weren't even aware we were experiencing any difficulties. My sister and her husband, David, knew all about our infertility problems, mainly because, well, we told them. We also spent more time with them than we did with our other friends. It is easy to put on a brave face for a few hours every now and again. It's harder when you spend every Sunday evening cooking and eating together. My sister and I have always been close, and her husband is one of Trent's friends from his time in Argentina. We have always made every opportunity to spend time together. I was sure that most people had not noticed the slow decline Trent and I were experiencing. Jessica and David saw the whole of it. She had been inviting us over even more often than usual. She even extended an open dinner invitation.

"Come over anytime. I don't need more than a few minutes warning. We'll feed you, and we'll have a great time."

"We'd love to have you," David added.

At the time, she was only twenty years old and a newlywed to boot. Both of them were students and as poor as, if not poorer than, Trent and I. Her offer to open up her home at a moment's notice was sincere and generous, especially for someone her age and in her circumstances. I realized she offered partly because of our fertility struggles. I knew she and her husband understood our situation better than most people. In fact, other than our parents, she and David were the ones who knew the most about our fertility troubles. They were eye witnesses to the some of the times we returned with disappointing news from the doctor's office. They knew a fair amount about the steps we were taking towards treatment.

Even though I knew they were privy to so many details, it shocked me to realize the depth of their worry for us. When Jessica asked if Trent was okay, I saw that she realized the seriousness of our trial, and she was seeing warning signs.

"I think he's just been upset about all the fertility stuff," I said.

Even then, with the knowledge that she understood the depth of our sorrow, I couldn't let the façade fall all the way. She didn't press. Neither did her husband. They just reminded us to come back anytime.

"We like you guys," they said.

When I talked to Trent about it, we came to the realization that we had been cloistering ourselves away. Sure, we spent time with family, but other than that, we spent little time socializing. We came to the conclusion that we did not want to disappear into disappointment. Too many victims drown in their own personal disasters. We didn't want to join the fallen.

We decided that, yes, we still needed to focus our efforts on fertility treatment. However, we needed to fill the spaces in between treatments. We needed to become more than the reflection of a far off and difficult dream.

Trent and I have always been borderline goofy. Even in our most serious moments, we'll make a wry comment or crack a joke. Since the diagnosis, our moments of levity came in shorter, weaker spurts. Realizing this, we decided to make a concerted effort to bring those moments back into greater prominence. We would watch a funny TV show or a video clip. We'd read funny stories. We'd tell jokes. We tried to tell puns. Anyone who watched this slow step in our recovery might have shaken their heads at us. We laughed long and hard at weak jokes. For us, the feeling of mirth felt so glorious, even liberating.

I feel like so many people try too hard to jump right back into their normal lives after having a catastrophic emotional event, acting as though nothing has changed. Like athletes who break their leg, the emotionally injured miss the way things used to be so much, they try to sprint before they are able. I don't mean to say that the emotionally injured's capacity for happiness remains forever altered. I mean that they need to take care of themselves. They need to exercise their emotional muscles with patience. Forcing feelings to come can cause frustration and disappointment.

We chose laughter as our first focus because it was an atrophied part of our personalities. It was also a fortuitous choice, medically speaking. The laughter helped us to produce endorphins. Endorphins help create energy and happiness. With our endorphin levels on the rise, we began to have a better overall mood. After months of incremental increases in our humor, I found I could even joke with the doctor while my feet were held in the much-hated stirrups. I've even made the nurses laugh a few times. It's an accomplishment I relish.

We turned then to books—not just fertility books, but genre fiction and great works of literary fiction. We listened to them as audiobooks together. Sometimes, on lazy Sunday afternoons, we would sprawl on the couches and listen for hours. We've always loved books, and returning to them felt like returning to an old friend. We even began to share our childhood favorites with each other and then hold long discussions.

We went back to taking long walks together. I got more involved in the writing community again. Trent started a more rigorous exercise routine. We traveled to visit our families for longer expanses of time.

The days of happiness stretched. Our capacity for happiness increased, and our abilities increased as well. Trent and I suffer from infertility, but if you take a look at how we live our lives, our struggle won't be the only priority that defines us. It's true that we are still trying with all our might to get pregnant. We are still frugal to the point of being cheap. We still try to plan our trips so that we don't miss any opportunities for treatment. But if you look closely, you will also see Trent as a devoted husband, a promising future dentist, an athlete, a singer, and an avid reader. You will see me as devoted wife, a writer, a singer, a budding Zumba enthusiast, and a good cook. Those stretched days of happiness have filled us up, until it is the days of sadness and struggle that are the days in between.

In Between

Every now and again, I forget that life is still good.
That chocolate still melts on the tongue,
that fall still burns red, yellow, and orange.
Riding my bike still brings quick-drying sweat,
and during long walks, my husband still holds my hand.

There are days that are dim or foggy;
there are days with icy roads.

But these are the days in between.
And the shadow they cast is only
a dark blotch on an otherwise vibrant painting.

PART TEN

TO ALL
THINGS
THERE IS A
SEASON

Decisions

When we found out we would need intense treatment in order to have children, Trent and I knew we were beginning a time of emotion-driven hurricanes as physically damaging as earthquakes. More than that, we realized that we would need to make significant, even difficult decisions. We knew we would need to make budgeting choices, decide when to go through certain procedures, and pick a time at which we would stop treatment and opt for adoption. But even homes with hurricane windows suffer broken glass, and even earthquake-proof buildings sometimes suffer damage when the quake hits. Despite all our efforts to anticipate what we would face, we weren't prepared for the complex moral choices we would encounter.

Trent and I are religious people. We pattern our lives to be faithful to the precepts taught by our church. Ideals like the sanctity of life, fidelity in marriage, and the importance of family are of supreme importance to us. When we began preparing for in vitro, we felt our treatment plan helped us in our efforts to follow those precepts. We still believe in vitro helps us in our goal; however, we didn't realize that the process would also force us to face those precepts. We didn't know we would need to think of those ideals in practical and complicated ways.

The truth about infertility is this: There will be moments when you will have to look at life and make godlike decisions. There will be times when you grant or revoke permission to create life or to destroy it. And despite having a very mortal mind, you will need to decide which of those godlike choices is heavenly and which is not. It may surprise you how hard it is to see the difference. The moment of our first godlike decision was triggered by a seemingly benign suspicion.

It began the first time we were preparing for in vitro. The doctor suggested that we get tested to see if we were carriers for any genetic diseases. He suspected that our particular type of infertility arose from a genetic defect—one that we could pass to our children. The doctor thought that, other than our infertility problems, we were asymptomatic carriers. But our children might be more than just carriers if both Trent and I carried the same genetic disease. They might inherit it.

"We'll test you for all the common types of genetic diseases. Even if one of you is a carrier of one defect, it's unlikely both of you will be. If it turns out both of you are carriers, we can screen the embryos before implantation. If any of the embryos turn up positive for the condition, we can decide what to do from there."

It took thirty seconds to see the full implications of the doctor's speech. We could destroy the embryos if we wanted to avoid having a baby with a genetic mutation. My reaction surprised me. Before we knew about the possibility of testing the baby before implantation, we made a decision that we would carry any and every baby to term. If the baby had genetic mutations, deformations, retardations, gestational defects, or any other abnormality, we would maintain the pregnancy and raise the child to the best of our ability.

We made that decision during a time when we thought there would be no way we could know about a problem until after the pregnancy began. The fact that we would now know about defects before the embryo transfer made me feel more responsibility for our child's quality of life. If we implanted an affected embryo in the full knowledge of all that implied, wouldn't any consequences be our fault?

Without question, neither Trent nor I wanted to use in vitro to select the perfect child. However, when we saw the list of possible genetic defects, I felt horrified. It frightened me to see the types of things we could pass to our child if we were found to be carriers. My husband, who is training to be a dentist, was learning about birth defects and genetic diseases that year.

I asked if he would tell me about them. He showed me the slides provided for the class. Some of the defects caused the lungs to be constantly filled with thick, plugging mucus. Some promised chronic infections. Others caused muscle degeneration. Some caused severe mental handicaps. Others significantly shortened lifespans. Worst were the ones that caused horrific, lifelong pain. I looked at the symptoms and imagined putting a child through that kind of gauntlet. I wondered if I could ever knowingly condemn a child to such a difficult life. Then I wondered if I could ever knowingly deny a child a chance at life, no matter how difficult or painful that life might be. If both Trent and I were carriers, and if we produced any embryos with genetic diseases, what would we do?

Some might say we should not have worried until after we knew more. Perhaps they would be right. In hindsight, I don't know if we should have considered the implications that early. I just know that I almost always want to make decisions when I can still take the time to consider all the implications of what I am choosing. When I was little, I decided I wouldn't use drugs or alcohol a decade before I was ever offered a cigarette or beer. As a teenager, I decided I would abstain from sex until marriage. I made that decision years before I even kissed a boy. Our tests would take a few weeks to yield results. To me, that already seemed a condensed time frame.

Trent and I tried to talk it out on our own. Before this, our choices took time, effort, and sometimes tears, but we always arrived at a course of action. This time, we talked over a few possibilities. We discussed not implanting the embryos and leaving them frozen. We didn't see a real difference between that and destroying them. We thought about not testing the embryos at all. Then we could spend up to nine months not knowing if our child would need extra care. We talked about implanting all the embryos regardless of any defects. We wondered if we could live with ourselves knowing we could have prevented their pain. We discussed abandoning in vitro in favor of adoption. Although we think we will someday adopt (even if in vitro works for us), the timing did not feel right.

Around this time, I talked to one of my friends who had already gone through the in vitro process. I asked her advice on how to handle everything, from needles to tests to passing time during the two weeks after in vitro in which no pregnancy test will be accurate. I didn't mention the genetic test. I didn't even know how to bring it up. She, however, mentioned the fact that she knew there would be a lot of moral choices put in front of us, and soon.

"Honestly," I said, "I'm beginning to think we might just wing it."

"That's always an option," she said, "but, in the spirit of full disclosure, you need to know that during this process, you will be pumped full of hormones. My advice would be to make all the decisions you can now, before your senses are clouded by hormones and stress."

After that conversation, Trent and I came to the conclusion that we needed some sort of outside help. The pressure of deific decision weighed down on us—making us feel smaller even than we were. I've seen people struggling with burdens like these: mothers of critically ill children, politicians with impossible dilemmas, and others who, like us, suffer infertility. Because none of us are gods, none of us should try to face these moments alone. Trent and I sought help, and when we did, we again turned to our minister for advice. We had moved since the last time we'd talked to a minister, so just like we had needed to change doctors, we had changed ministers as well. We explained our situation; then we told him about the genetic test and how we weren't sure what to do. We asked for his theological counsel. Even he looked flummoxed. He asked if he could take us to a private room to ask more detailed questions. We agreed.

He asked questions with gentle thoroughness, explaining that he just wanted to get a better picture of our situation. He'd never been asked about it before and wanted to give accurate, well-informed advice.

"Would it be an egg or sperm or fertilized embryo?"

"A fertilized embryo."

"Would the embryo already be developing inside you?"

"No."

"Does every embryo need to be implanted?"

"No."

"Is it possible that you won't get pregnant even after the embryo is transferred?"

"Yes."

"Would they be able to tell for sure if the embryo is affected?"

"The test is pretty accurate, but not infallible."

Our minister sat there, head resting on his hand, eyes unfocused as he considered our answers. He took out an ecclesiastical manual of instruction and read for a moment. With a sigh, he turned back to us.

"I don't know," he said. "I honestly don't know what to say. Is it alright if I consult a minister of higher authority?"

We told him we would appreciate that. In some ways, we felt vindicated in our uncertainty. We were facing a decision difficult enough to cause even our minister to pause and think. In other ways, we were worried. What if no one knew what to tell us, or what if the advice came too late? In the meantime, we took the test. We could have opted not to take the test; however, we felt strongly that we should proceed at least that far.

Before our minister found the theological standard of our church, we received the test results. We both tested negative for the entire gamut of genetic diseases. The test is not infallible; no medical test is. Even knowing that, we felt our fears ease. We might still give birth to a child with handicaps or other difficulties, but we no longer need to wonder what to do. We've already decided to maintain the pregnancy and raise any child, no matter what.

We let our minister know that we no longer needed to know our church's official stance on the issue. When he asked if we still wanted him to check, we said no. I hope it doesn't seem like cowardice, but we decided that since the need to choose was mercifully taken from us, we would not even try to decide. We would save our energy for the next heartbreaking choice.

Though we were spared the need to decide if we would implant embryos affected by a genetic mutation, we still face more choices. There's the chance, however slim, that we might produce more embryos than we ever want to use. We like children, but I can't see us being the parents of twenty or more. If we do have too many, we need to decide what to do with the remainder. Do we keep them in reserve, just in case? Do we donate them to other infertile couples? Do we donate them to science? Do we destroy them?

There is also the chance that both of us could die before using all our embryos. At one clinic, we were asked to sign paperwork to designate a guardian for any un-implanted children. Even before they are twenty cells old, we need to ensure our kids are taken care of. Of course, those guardians will need to be told what our wishes for the embryos would be. If we don't, we leave them with the dilemma of what to do if we pass on. It's a strange feeling, making a decision for someone who isn't yet there. We hadn't even made any embryos yet, and we were signing paperwork that would affect them. It's like we are parents of phantoms and half-made promises. The strangest part is that as diaphanous and vague as these half-made promises are, I feel an obligation to them. I want to give them the safety that only a parent can offer. And I felt somehow comforted that I might be able to offer even this much possible protection.

Even after the godlike decisions end, mortal considerations come up that, though not as daunting, can still overwhelm. For us, just the sheer magnitude of the menial mortal decisions added considerable emotional pressure. For example, we also needed to decide when enough is enough. Even in vitro is not a guarantee. At some point, we may need to decide to stop. We have looked at how far our finances might stretch. We've tried to guess how much stress in vitro might put on our bodies. We've tried to imagine the emotional stress. We've decided on a few possible stopping points. I won't say what they are. There is no moral marker for in vitro endurance.

Then, once we try to stop in vitro, we need to decide what to do next. If I'm never able to get pregnant or never able to carry a child to term, we need to decide what option to take. Do we want to try adoption right away or take some time to grieve? One of my friends even volunteered to be our surrogate if we ever decided we wanted to pursue that route. Even with that amazing offer, we would need to decide if we could accept such an incredible sacrifice. And if we did decide to accept, how would we make the process as comfortable as possible for her?

We've come to most of our decisions. It has taken time, effort, (in our case) prayer, and more than a little guess work. I imagine as we continue with the process and gather more information, we may need to re-evaluate our conclusions, pray some more, and guess some more.

I won't reveal our choices in this book. It's not that either Trent or I are ashamed of our choices. Rather, I prefer not to say because I don't want to influence anyone else. There is just so much to consider: the price of treatment, the emotional toll, the moral ramifications, and the prognosis for treatment. Every choice is highly individual. All I feel like I can advise is that whatever decisions a couple makes, they make it together. These choices are too heavy to bear alone.

Time

ime is that ever-present mocker of those suffering infertility. A woman is born with a limited number of eggs. Every month, she loses more. Men begin to lose their virility as they age. They produce fewer sperm, and the sperm they do produce are of lesser quality and vitality. Our thirties are still years away, but my husband and I worry that we will not have as many children as we want because we may run out of time. We need to invest time and money, both of which are difficult to come by, especially now.

There are other things in life we want. We want to travel. We want to be able to buy a house. We want to drive a better car—the kind that doesn't break down at least twice a year. We don't mind waiting for those things. Europe will still be there for us to visit whether we are twenty-five or eighty-five. I've never known a time where there were no homes on the market. Cars get made by the thousands every year.

Eventually, Trent and I will have nothing left to give toward becoming biological parents. Time has never felt so precious, nor moved so quickly. My deadline comes much more quickly than Trent's. For women, the drop-off in fertility comes right at age thirty-five. People with normal fertility levels can get pregnant long past then, sure. But for those of us already having a hard time of it, thirty-five is a frightening number. It's not an absolute deadline, but it is the start of new and significant obstacles. When those obstacles are combined with the first, they might become insurmountable.

It's such an odd thing to think that I am in a race against my own body. Losing means I've thwarted myself.

Timing

When infertility strikes, couples need to brace themselves for a ride with sprints and stops—a rollercoaster with amazing climbs, drops, and sudden, complete inertial arrests. Before I began this journey, I never thought how pliable time could be, how much and how little control we have over its passing. More than that, I didn't know just how much more difficult time management would become when suddenly there were so many parties struggling to control that timeline: me, my husband, my unborn children, and (as I believe) God. It's a rollercoaster and a wrestling match where sometimes the only form of control is surrender, the only way to show love is through sacrifice, and the only way to persevere is sheer stubbornness. Many assume that this strange vortex begins at the moment infertility is diagnosed. That's not the case. The journey begins the moment that future parents begin discussing that inciting question: "When?"

After a few weeks of being engaged, we began talking about when to have children. Like so many others, we had no idea we were infertile. Trent wanted a honeymoon baby; I wanted to wait one year before trying for children. Both of us wanted children, wanted them with the conviction of those who believe that parenthood is the highest calling in life. You wouldn't think

a year would be much cause for discussion. We could compromise at six months. We could decide not to compromise at
all; it's only a year's difference. But we both had significant and
pressing reasons for our timetables.

In those days, in order to have privacy, we took long walks,
often in the evening. During a cold fall dusk, we discussed when
to start expanding our family.

We didn't fight. Fighting involves anger and malicious intent.
We weren't angry, but we were in direct and determined opposi-
tion to the other's time frame. We considered our words. There
were a lot of words to be shared, worries and hopes to be confided, disappointments to be expressed, and practical realities
to be faced. We went over budgeting numbers, insurance plans,
graduation dates, and health concerns. In the end, we decided
that we would wait a year.

In my own words, "I think waiting a year would be best. But
longer than a year? That would be just too long to wait for children."

To say that Trent wasn't disappointed or upset would be a
lie. I think he was very disappointed. Trent is a laser-focused
person. Once he zeroes in on the apparent task, he finishes it and
moves on to the next task. He had found me and dated me until
he knew he wanted to marry me. In a few months, we would
be married. The next obvious task after marriage seemed inevitable: begin expanding our family. When we decided to delay,
it was a sacrifice on his part, and not just because he wanted a
child. He sacrificed the general inertia of his life's course. That
loss of inertia is difficult for a laser.

We waited that year. It's strange to think that we were infertile even then. We had no idea that we didn't need the birth control. We didn't know that the year we had set aside for ourselves would have come and gone with or without our choice to wait. When we started trying, we were both on the same page. Each of us felt ready for pregnancy to begin at any moment. We watched for signs. Looking back, it was a ridiculous performance. A backache, a sour stomach, or a mood swing sent me running to buy a pregnancy test. If sheer wanting could have made me pregnant, I would be the mother of several sets of triplets by now.

People often imagine that husband and wife have identical desires of when and how to treat infertility, especially when both want to be treated. It seems logical that they want every test done as soon as it can be done. In most cases, couples don't go in for infertility treatments unless they are both ready to become parents. Trent and I weren't any different from the norm. By the time we sought treatment, we both showed signs of the stress and worry.

What people don't understand is that so much more goes into the decision to receive each different fertility treatment. The first item to consider is that fertility treatments are expensive and almost never covered by insurance companies. Then, diagnostic testing can reveal embarrassing bodily abnormalities. And not every person has the same odds of having treatment be successful. Your own body can grow weak and tired from the changes in hormones or the pregnancy losses. Certain treatments involve finding donors or surrogates, and treatments are often unromantic and stressful. Further, couples must often make complex moral decisions before proceeding with a treatment. I could go on.

These are real-world detriments and they cause real-life disagreements. A husband may refuse to submit to a semen analysis. A wife might refuse to go in for an appointment that is sure to include yet another pelvic exam. Couples can disagree on how much they are willing to spend on treatments. One spouse might decide the emotional trauma takes too much of their energy, while the other is still desperate to try at least one more treatment. These conflicts of interest produce a temporal friction. Time still moves, but now the couple feels its passage over their minds and skin. The constant discomfort and friction caused by disagreement can sometimes spark marital conflict. For us, the lack of romance and the shame of needing treatment caused just such a spark.

I remember the inciting incident came after one of the rare doctor's appointments where I went to the doctor without Trent. I came home telling my husband about a great treatment option for us: an Intrauterine Insemination (IUI). The treatment is not very expensive and even less invasive. Once the woman ovulates, the man gives a semen sample and the sample is put into the woman's uterus via a catheter. I explained this to Trent. Trent does not hide his emotions well. I felt my happiness fade as his face slid from a smile to a look of distress. I asked him what was wrong.

I was more than willing to overlook the utilitarian process of an IUI in order to gain the results. Trent was not. With frankness (but not rudeness), he confided his concerns. He saw the complete and utter lack of romance in the procedure. The blatant lack of love during the conception process set his teeth on edge. He wanted to wait.

I told him, with equal frankness, the procedure's lack of romance made no difference to me. I told him I thought we might be able to invent some sort of romance to accompany the unwieldy process. I wanted to move forward. The opportunity seemed too good to turn down. He nodded, but his eyes never met mine. For Trent, lack of eye contact means disagreement and/or discontent.

I sighed and asked him, "If it worked, would you be disappointed? Is it possible you would regret the pregnancy?"

"I'm not sure," he said. "Maybe. It's possible."

Then he told me something else that surprised me. He confessed that he might feel like he had not fathered the child. Please do not misunderstand. Trent was not implying he would feel as if I had been unfaithful to him. He felt that the necessity for so much interference by medicine and so little lovemaking would strip him of any responsibility for good results. It would be his sperm and my egg, yes, but it would be a syringe, a catheter, and a doctor who would get me pregnant, not him.

Timing fertility treatments would be so much easier if time were the only priority. Or even if it were only about time and money. Money can be earned, and fertility doctors are great at responding to a couple's sense of urgency. But time and money are not the only factors. More emotional needs often shift timetables. In this instance, it was my husband who needed time to halt. The intense feelings facing him needed time to play out, to heal, and to come to some resolution. We decided to wait. But, of course, it wasn't only my husband who needed time to heal. I did, too, but I didn't need time to slow down; I needed it to speed up.

My breakdown came Christmas day. We were spending the school break with Trent's family. I knew I was pregnant. I just knew it. My breasts were sore, and my stomach bubbled and tossed. After Christmas dinner, my stomach started to boil in earnest. I ran upstairs just in time to throw up. Never before had I felt so much triumph while puking into a toilet bowl. I knew that, this time, I was pregnant! Then, a few hours later, my period started. So did a fever. I was disappointed. I was angry. I was on my period. I was throwing up. And it was Christmastime.

Fleeing the indignity and sadness, I retreated to the room we had been given for our stay. I didn't want to tell anyone the exact depth of my disappointment. Trent and I were still keeping our infertility quiet. We hoped that our trial would be short-lived, and we didn't want to worry anyone over a passing misfortune. Despite our lingering hope, I felt quite certain we would need medical interference. Sensing we would need help, knowing that Trent wasn't ready to receive help, and feeling so disappointed at yet another failure, I started to cry.

"I just kept thinking how perfect it would be," I said to Trent, "to announce a pregnancy during Christmas break."

"I know," he said, running his fingers through my sweaty hair.

"It will be the same next month, you know," I said. "I won't be pregnant next month, either."

"What makes you so sure? You might get pregnant. You never know."

The more miserable I am, the harder it is for me to not get upset, to not lash out. I tried so hard to not say anything hurtful, but I also wanted . . . no, I needed to tell him the strength of my unhappiness. Trying to push past all the horrible emotions, I opened my mouth to explain. The words came out of me like oil pressed from olives: slow and dripping.

"Because. What . . . on earth . . . will be different from this month to next? There's something wrong. Unless that something changes, I will not get pregnant."

I was asking him to give the okay for us to try an IUI. I was asking without asking. I wanted it all so badly. I already felt like my failure to get pregnant reflected poorly on my femininity. My confidence was broken and rattling inside of me. Of course, not only my confidence was broken. Trent felt that his inability to get me pregnant reflected poorly on his masculinity. If I got pregnant with an IUI, my problem would be solved. Not his.

And because my problem could be eventually resolved, and his could not, we waited several more months. Timing is like that. Despite the fact that couples who face infertility both have the same goal in mind, each has a slightly different clicking clock in the brain. Deciding which to follow can cause strife. For us, we decided that we would switch back and forth between the clocks according to whose need was greater.

Time made our joint desperation grow deep enough that Trent reconciled himself to the necessity of the procedure. On the day we went in to perform the IUI, the doctor ran a quick check on both of us to make sure we were ready for the procedure. After the results came in, we were told that the IUI would be all but pointless. We would need to move on to in vitro. Trent and I sat there in complete silence.

We were students. In vitro can cost as much as twenty thousand dollars just to get pregnant. The labor and delivery would be up to ten thousand more. At that time, our combined income came nowhere near thirty thousand. Our quest for parenthood had to wait. Again. It was the first time that timing would be wrenched from our hands. We no longer decided when and where and how. Our finances and doctors' recommendations did.

During all this time, I had been having difficult menstrual cycles. I often felt so much pain that I would be incapacitated for days. After we were told we would need to do in vitro, Trent came to me and suggested I talk to the doctor about going back on the pill for pain management. If we couldn't get pregnant without in vitro, maybe I should take the pill, controlling the physical pain until we could move forward with other treatments. I went in to my doctor. I described the pain I often experienced and then explained how I wouldn't ask to go back on the pill if I felt like I could manage the pain. He wrote me a prescription on the spot.

"Take it," he said. "Not taking it would be pointless suffering on your part. Take it, and don't feel guilty."

Up to that point, doctors and nurses and medical assistants had all advised us to continue to try for children.

"It only takes one egg and one sperm," they said, as if it were a slogan.

I went home, and before filling the prescription, told Trent what the doctor had said. It was a strange and sad relief. I've never been so disappointed but so glad at the same time. Each month, as the cycle restarted, I spent up to a full week feeling punished for the fact that I was not pregnant. At times, I'd even begin to wonder if it was a judgment from heaven, a slight variation from Eve's. *I will greatly multiply thy sorrow but eliminate thy conception; in sorrow thou shalt not bring forth children.*

Trent knew and understood my feelings. We were unanimous in our grief that even the doctors had stopped urging us to allow hope for the one egg and one sperm. Strange how that slogan had been such an annoying bolster. I think many who suffer infertility understand that feeling: the hope of others both sets you afloat and chafes at you. It's like an ill-fitting life preserver. You want to believe they are right—that everything can be just fine. The thought that they might be wrong rubs you raw. We were also unanimous in our relief that at least waiting would not be so physically painful for me.

We filled the prescription that day. Medical doctors would argue that, from that point until the point I would decide to go off of birth control, Trent and I were no longer trying for children. From a medical perspective, I can see their point. I don't agree with them, however. I've known other couples who have halted treatments to earn money. Women who have gone back on birth control after miscarriages, to let their body heal. I've known men who had corrective surgeries that required them to refrain from intimacy for a time. All of these people—all of us—were working towards having children, trying for them, but through means other than intercourse. For Trent and I, we saved all the money we could. Our timetable now depended on how much we could save. Our means to children was no longer eggs and sperm, but dollars and cents. We waited and saved. We spent our time living as much as possible on as little as possible. Living has a way of bringing you back to yourself. For a long time, we had been defined by our struggle for children. Living life, even with the caveat of saving for something more, felt like a healing balm. We never worried about taking a pregnancy test. We just knew the answer: no. The sole question we worried about was when we would have enough money to start in vitro.

After several months of saving, we received an offer of help that would enable us to begin treatments sooner than we anticipated. Because we had moved, we found a new fertility doctor and scheduled an initial consultation. After reviewing our history, he told us that he put our chances of conceiving at 45 percent with one cycle and 90 percent with four. I sat stunned. For the first time in forever, someone was speaking to us with optimism about our chances for having a child. When we told him we needed another three months before starting a cycle, he made a suggestion.

Often, during fertility treatments, someone puts forth a sort of gamble treatment—a solution that just might shorten all the suffering and anguish. These treatments come with different costs in different currencies, but always included in the price is time.

He knew of another treatment option we could test: a certain type of vitamin might help raise fertility levels. It worked for about 5 percent of the people who tried, but the treatment cost so little and required no doctor. We didn't even need a prescription. Five percent is dismal. In one hundred people, only five have any success. Still, in a million people, fifty thousand have success. It sounds more promising, but the proportion is the same. On the way home, the sound of it became euphonious. A chance. A chance to maybe get pregnant without spending thousands of dollars to get pregnant; it felt like an offer of paradise.

We weren't just thinking of our first child either. If we could conceive without in vitro this first time, we might be able to do it again. We had been planning to do in vitro with every child. With us wanting six children, and with the price being around twenty thousand dollars each time, it would mean spending a total of one hundred and twenty thousand dollars. Children are priceless; in vitro is expensive.

Then came the cacophonous note. As part of the means of testing the success of the fertility vitamins, I would need to go off of the pill. I did not want to go back to those painful times. On top of that, I dreaded the wondering and the wanting. Just the idea of being able to have children without in vitro cooed at me. I knew that if we tried, I would stare that 5 percent in the face and spend a whole month aching and hoping to be one of the lucky few who make up that statistic, convinced it would be us. I did not want to try for such a long shot. I knew Trent wanted to try. Again, our timetables were in conflict.

We made the decision at our apartment complex pool. In a way, the setting felt nostalgic. We were making a major choice outdoors again. It was the middle of a weekday and no one came in to swim. I started to talk. I reminded him of all the days I had spent in pain. I told him how I did not want to expend so much hope on a long shot. I didn't know if I could handle going back to so much pain and hope all at once, especially since it would more than likely be in vain.

Trent did remember the times I'd been in pain. He always took care of me as best as he could, keeping track of when I'd taken pain killers, making all the meals, and doing all of the chores while I couldn't move. And he remembered how much it had hurt me to face disappointment after hope. He had always been there to hold me when I cried. He could have reminded me of all the times he'd been there for me. He could have used that as leverage toward getting what he wanted.

Instead, he reminded me of the IUI, and how he had felt cheated. He reminded me how he had felt like, if it had worked, he would not be the one to get me pregnant. He had, after growing desperate, decided to try the procedure because the desire to have a child had become so great and so urgent. He would not regret the procedure or any pregnancy that would result, regardless of the pain it caused him. The necessity of the procedure saddened him, but that regret could not be undone. In fact, with in vitro, his regret had deepened. The process had now become even further removed from either of us. Our success at having children would rely more on our doctors' skill than our love, with more need of needles and catheters than romance. At least, it seemed that way. Now, we had an opportunity to get everything back: romance, pride, and normalcy. He knew he cared more about that opportunity than I did. He knew, in many ways, this opportunity would be hell for me.

He asked, "Could you do it? Could you do it for me?"

It isn't very often that we are offered the chance to take someone else's suffering on ourselves. Trent never asked me to go to hell all alone. He asked me to try and rescue him from a hell he'd long ago accepted for himself.

When Trent is sick, I can't take the fever. When Trent is struggling with work or school, I can't take his workload. I wish I could. There have been times I prayed that I could take some of Trent's pain onto myself.

At the moment Trent asked me to save him from hell; I didn't realize the greatness of the gift given to me. I only saw the pain like a red-hot thing in my mind. I saw the soiled hope like a gray cloud, pressing next to the pain. I was afraid, and I didn't want to try. I've come to realize that pain doesn't feel real until it is right there in front of you. All the times I had asked to take Trent's pain, I had been willing but naive.

I could see all the real red and gray pain. I also saw Trent. He already faced significant pain, and I knew it, and I didn't want him to be in pain anymore. My decision carried the power to give him a chance at relief. Despite my misgivings, despite my reluctance, the time Trent asked me save him from hell, I said yes.

Before continuing with the story, I want to stress that Trent never asked me to risk my health. The pain was real, yes, but it was just that: pain. The pill helped regulate my pain, nothing more. Trent never has put my health at risk, nor will he. I did go off the pill, and the pain did come. Though I regret the necessity, I cannot regret the decision.

I am not sure how many of us were trying the same treatment at the same time. If there were one hundred of us, about five got happy news. If there were a million of us, about fifty thousand got that news. I am happy for them, and I'm jealous. Trent and I were not part of that 5 percent. The treatment had made no difference at all in our prognosis. We began to prepare for in vitro.

Our next step was more practical and sure than the gamble we had just taken. We had high hopes for its success. But sometimes timing gets wrenched by a completely random source from the hands of planners. Life contains so many different timelines, and though they might often seem like they run parallel to each other, they often times collide. Our collision caused a temporary derailment. During the planning, an old health problem began to resurface. I tried to put it out of my mind. I tried to push it away as nothing. After a while, I could no longer deny it: my right side needed treatment.

About a year before we started preparing for in vitro, my upper-right side had begun to burn with a constant, dull ache. After a few months of it not getting worse, but not getting better, Trent and I went in to the doctor. The placement of the ache made doctors suspicious of gallbladder disease. They sent me in for an ultrasound, but the results came back normal.

When I told the doctor how Trent and I had recently discovered how difficult it would be for us to have children, he asked me if that had caused any stress.

If I'm not expecting the question, I am not very good at

saying exactly what I feel the moment someone asks me, especially if I feel like they should be able to get some sort of idea of what I am feeling just from context. To me, the doctor asking if the discovery of the depth of our infertility made me stressed equated to asking the victim of a plane crash if they felt a bit shaken. All of what I could have said about how neither Trent nor I could sleep well, about how socializing required unusual amounts of energy, about how I felt like my life was irrevocably changed, built up in my mind and got stuck.

"Yes," I said.

The doctor sent me home with a powerful antacid. He thought it might be an ulcer. I took the antacid and some of my symptoms seemed to ameliorate, so I didn't go back to the doctor. As the year passed, the ache would come and go. My father told me to keep track of when my symptoms returned, and to check if it got worse after eating either spicy or fatty foods. I kept track. No foods triggered any change whatsoever. The only consistency seemed to be that it always accompanied a sudden increase in stress. As the dull ache ebbed away to almost nothing, I started to feel like the problem resolved itself.

Fast forward to the time we decided to go ahead with in vitro. Though excited by our new opportunity, some aspects of the process caused a new spike in stress. Needles petrify me. I had already given vial after vial of blood for tests. Each test put me through the same ordeal. Trent holds one hand, already slick with sweat, while the nurse sticks the opposite arm. Then the shaking starts. Slow clamminess spreads from my fingers then settles in my elbows. My head seems to drain of fluid and fill with cotton. In the minute or less it takes to give blood, I turn into a tight-lipped wreck.

In vitro meant more tests. In vitro meant needles every day for the whole egg-ripening process. We went to a class to prepare us for the procedure ahead, and we learned a great deal. The most likely complication from in vitro is twins. The other possible complications are highly unlikely, especially for a young and healthy person. Often, those complications can come with normal pregnancies, anyway. As the instructor told us about hyper-stimulation and ectopic pregnancies, I felt myself enter an hour-long episode of lightheaded discomfort.

Then the talk of pricing came. The medicine for in vitro was not included in the package we were considering. We needed to pay several thousand dollars more than what we expected. The combined prices added up to as much as buying a new car.

Then we were given needles to practice mixing the medicines and filling syringes. They kept exclaiming over the small size of the needles. I don't look at the needles nurses use to take my blood. I look away. At the class, I didn't just look at the needles. I handled them, pressed the syringe levers up and down, felt how much resistance there would be as either Trent or I plunged liquid hormones under my skin. I could see and touch the piece of metal that would go into me every night for days.

My side began to burn again. It kept me awake at night. I worried that perhaps the problem would be a risk to any pregnancy. Two weeks before in vitro, I told Trent I needed the doctor. Trent went with me. We had moved since the last time I'd gone in to complain about my side. I had to explain things to the new doctor. After the exam, the doctor told me I would need to do some tests and that, in the meantime, I should cancel in vitro.

A doctor is not God. Neither Trent nor I took his word as gospel. We talked about it. I was worried. I was worried that I might have gallbladder disease, and I didn't want to take care of gallbladder disease in the midst of a pregnancy. It would be dangerous for me and the baby. I told Trent that my stomach felt so full of pressure and achiness, I couldn't imagine fitting a baby in the same general area. And if I did get pregnant, what would happen if the baby kicked the sore spot in my side? I also admitted that I worried the pain might all be in my head. I worried that we would spend money we needed for in vitro on a medical goose chase.

It was two weeks before in vitro. We had made all sorts of plans for the procedure. If we decided to delay, we might be forced to retake expensive and uncomfortable tests. Most pre–in vitro tests need to be redone every six months. We might even need to select a different in vitro plan—which might cost several thousand dollars more. Our insurance deductible reached well over five thousand dollars, so we would pay for all of the diagnostic testing. Without hesitation, Trent told me he wanted me to find out the source of the problem, and that I should not feel guilty about investigating. When we told the fertility doctor, he too advised prompt investigation.

In the end, we found that all the stress of our situation caused my digestion to slow and become inefficient. The doctor advised de-stressing (oh, how simple that sounds). The knowledge that

I suffered from hyper-stressed guts, and not gallbladder disease or cancer or some other significant ailment, helped.

In the end, we did need to evaluate our decision for in vitro. We waited for my stomach to start feeling better, just to make sure de-stressing would take care of the problem. Waiting meant repeated tests, just like we knew it would. Waiting meant re-planning our budget. Waiting meant more time without a child.

During that time, I found another office that offered in vitro with less medication, which meant less cost, and less stress. Our previous doctor had been very good, but we decided to switch to the office that offered the different form of in vitro. The time we took to relax and make the change in treatment did the trick. I began to feel better.

We are still waiting for children. We still need to make decisions about timing. Trent has asked me for tremendous physical sacrifice. I have asked Trent for tremendous emotional sacrifice. Neither of us could have asked for what we did from any other person. We would have had no right. As each other's spouses, we've made promises to love and cherish one another and sacrifice for each other. We've done that. We've done it again and again. We will continue to do it. Some people are torn to pieces by the sacrifices they are asked to make in the name of having children. Marriages are ripped into bitter tatters.

We were saved, but not by having a complete and unified idea of what or when everything should happen. Nor were we saved because of the abiding force of our eternal love. We survived because we acted on the promises we had made the day of our marriage. Now, as we look back on those sacrifices, we see them as blessings and opportunities to fulfill our promises to each other.

Long Lines

I used to sketch long-lined scenes
with jointed graphite strokes,
like the limbs of a giant stick bug.

My sidewalks stretched deep into the paper,
past the grotesquely tall
grocery stores, laundromats,
and bookshops stacked
on the left and right sides of the street,
even past the local parks I couldn't fit into the drawing
    proper.

My ocean scenes modeled horizons,
so distant the parallel lines ended only
at the vanishing point.
Impossible. Considering the Earth's
rounding and circumference.

As the years have passed,
my drawings have more curves,
and the subject matter seems closer
to the surface of the paper.
I'm not sure if that means my perspective has changed,
or if I'm closer to the things I want.

PART ELEVEN

LOVE
IN A TIME
OF TRIAL

Romance

Traditional in vitro begins with repression—then blood, not love. You take birth control pills and sometimes injections. Then, during the first three days of a menstrual cycle, you go into the doctor's office for an ultrasound. The doctor takes some measurements of the uterus and ovaries. He or she makes sure that everything looks normal. If it hasn't happened yet, you learn how to give yourself injections, how to mix medicines, how to time shots and appointments. Then the doctor sends you home with needles and powders and bottles of liquid and sometimes pills, too.

For about two weeks, you give yourself the injections. During this time, you go in for follow up appointments. Ultrasounds and/or blood work are required to help measure your ovaries' reaction to the medications. Your dosing may change. It might stay the same. The doctor then tells you what day to take your trigger shot.

The trigger shot ripens the eggs on your ovaries, preparing them for harvest. You must take it at a certain time of day. Take it too early, and the eggs may have launched themselves into the fallopian tubes where they will do you as much good as they have in the past. Take it too late, and the eggs will be unripe and unusable. Either way, late or early, the cycle can be a complete loss. So you take the shot on time. You set the alarms and ask a friend to call and remind you. You take it on time, because by now you have spent up to five thousand dollars on the medicine alone. This shot is intramuscular, so (unless you are very brave) your husband gives that to you. Right in the gluteus maximus.

On egg retrieval day, you and your husband both go in. He gives a semen sample, or, if he has a severe problem sperm count, motility, or morphology, he goes to a room where the doctor retrieves sperm directly from the testicles. You go into a room where the doctor uses an ultrasound-guided needle. The needle removes the eggs directly from the ovary. It's a mercy you are sedated when this happens. If your husband is having his sperm harvested, he has to face his own needle and is also sedated. The doctor fertilizes the eggs that day. It takes several days to find out how well the fertilization process worked.

If the fertilization process goes well, you go in to transfer the embryos. The doctor selects one or two (or, in rare cases, more) embryos that look the most promising. The embryos are placed in a catheter that resembles a long, thin straw with a syringe attached. The doctor inserts this catheter past the cervix and up into the uterus. Then he uses the syringe to propel the embryos. If you request, any remaining embryos are frozen for future use.

You need two or three days of taking it easy or bed rest. During this time, you take progesterone shots or suppositories to help maintain the pregnancy. You might or might not be pregnant. Because you have taken the trigger shot, any pregnancy test you take for approximately two weeks will show that you are pregnant, even if you are not. So you don't take a pregnancy test. After the waiting time has passed, you go in to get your blood drawn. You are either pregnant or not.

It's a miracle of modern science that this process is even possible. During this process, there is no love making while making a baby. Your husband is given a cup, or is stabbed by a needle. You are impregnated by a syringe with a straw. There's no romance, no courtship.

Before we had even considered in vitro, Trent and I attended an interesting class. The class curriculum focused on making a marriage better. It did not count for any sociology or psychology credits. It was not meant to be used to help counsel other married couples. Rather, we learned strategies to strengthen our own personal marriage. Some of the material repeated facts so often it felt like being bludgeoned. Some of the material made us laugh. Some, we applied to our marriage with religious fervor. One particular piece of advice stood out. The teacher encouraged us all to never abandon the courtship stage.

"Men, continue to date your wife. Women, continue to date your husband. Continue to make your spouse feel that they are worth being made a fuss over, that you enjoy spending time with them. Continue to have fun."

And so we do. We go on dates every week. Every single week. Sometimes the date may be as simple as walking in a park or a renting a movie. We hold hands and kiss, in public as well as private. We've even gotten compliments (I hope they are sincere) about how our kisses are cute. We love it. We love each other. We love being together. We love the fact that we have been married for years and yet we still go out and do fun things like ride ferris wheels, hike, go to movies, and go for walks. Sometimes we remember the days where all we had to think about for the future was what our wedding day would be like.

We always expected reality would catch up with us. We knew that careers would come, that schooling would last for years after we married. We knew there would be bills. We understood there would be sickness. We even realized there would be days we were angry with each other. We knew we would argue. We didn't know that one of the key elements of our romantic relationship might become a source of great stress.

The first few months of infertility testing didn't cause any romantic tension. When the testing just begins, the desperation hasn't hit yet. The treatment, too, is pretty lax.

"Just make sure to time intercourse to when your temperature and test strips say you are ovulating," the doctors say.

Some people recommend abstaining for a few days before your presumptive ovulation date. Sometimes we did that. Sometimes we didn't.

It's as the months start passing that you are put in real danger of making pregnancy and childbearing a higher priority than your marriage. You begin to consider a more structured sexual schedule. You start to reject romantic advances because you need to keep things in reserve. Then there is the day you must have intercourse, or risk missing the golden opportunity. And, since you are infertile, if you miss one, you might be missing the only one that would result in a full-term pregnancy and successful delivery.

Just as we were entering the time when these thoughts were

coming to our minds, the doctors started to take things more seriously, too. They asked us to do some more tests. One of those tests was a semen analysis.

Standard procedure for a semen analysis is that the man is given a sterile cup. He is then sent to the bathroom. He masturbates into the cup. The doctor collects the sample and evaluates several different aspects of the ejaculate. Our doctor suggested a different approach. When he handed the cup to my husband, instead of sending him to the bathroom, he told us to go home.

"To the best of your ability," he said, "make this a romantic experience. Take all the time you need. Come back when you are done. You two are trying to have a baby together. This should be romantic."

He gave us a few further instructions, then sent us home. We were so new to the experience we didn't realize something unusual had happened. We assumed this was standard advice for all couples experiencing infertility. It was such a small thing, but I see it now as a preemptive strike to save our marriage.

The treatments of infertility—the diagnostic testing, the need to regulate sex to a schedule, etc.—all of it seems to take all the love making out of making a baby. The only way to stop the descent into loveless sex is to know it is coming and to make the decision that there will be something to look forward to, that there will be love and happiness, even in the midst of such rigid guidelines.

The absolute details of romance should never be shared, and so I won't share them here. Suffice it to say, there are ways to show love, even when there are shots to be taken or given. There are ways to make love when giving a semen sample. There can be romance even when the act of making love only ever produces love, not children.

We're trying to have a baby. It's romantic. We make it romantic.

Disclaimer: Please note that the traditional in vitro process varies slightly from clinic to clinic. I have tried to describe the process generically, but if you are planning an in vitro cycle, please consult your doctor about the details of your procedure.

Giving of Hands

I offer up comfort from my hands:
twin consecrated tools given to me
by a God who crafted each
line in my palms.

I wasn't given the power to lay these hands,
as a priest lays them,
on my husband's head to speak promises
of what blessings will come.

I wasn't given the power to lay my
hands on my husband's head
to command his anxieties
and wounds to knit themselves away.

But I was given hands with power,
not like a priest, but like a priestess;
not like a God, but like a Goddess.
I take my husband: pain, wounds, heartache, and all;
I hold him in my hands until
his hurting slips through my fingers
and only he remains.

Prepared

I don't feel unique when I say that there was a time when the infertility started to shatter my confidence; like safety glass, I was broken, but retained my basic shape. I felt a deep, bone-weakening shock. Never had I imagined that it would be difficult for me to get pregnant. The longer we spent with no success, the more bewildered I felt. When it dawned on me that this trial would last the rest of our lives, the world locked into a state of perpetual wrongness. The continuous parade of doctors and disappointment seemed the most prominent additions to the new life. I felt resourceless against this new world—as vulnerable as shell-less turtle. As I often do when I'm feeling deep distress, I asked Trent for comfort and advice.

While praying together, Trent got the impression that I had been prepared for this trial. We were intended to endure this time of difficulty together. That idea took a moment for me to absorb. Me? Him? All my years growing up, I assumed my husband and I would be so fertile it would be difficult for me to keep from getting pregnant. All my teenage years I hoped I could marry young, so I could begin my family young. None of that seemed like preparation to me. And what about Trent? Trent spent his teenage years in conscientious preparation to become a wonderful husband and father. At as young as eighteen, he let people know how much he looked forward to starting a family. How had he, who spent even his teenage years focusing all his soul toward becoming a father, been prepared to wait years for children?

Despite my initial doubt, a feeling of warmth started just behind my breastbone, a sensation I have always associated with confirmation of truth. The confirmation came without any sort of outside influence. There were no evident signs that Trent and I were meant to go through this ordeal. Despite my reservations, some deep intuition told me he was right.

It has taken years for me to start to see the moments that lead up to where we are now. As the years have rolled forward, I find myself peeling the time backward to before we knew about our infertility. I can see in us the seeds of what made us strong enough to handle this situation. I can see the habits that gave us a wellspring of fortitude.

Trent and I met when we were eighteen years old. Looking back at old pictures of the two of us, I see two newborn adults. Our cheeks still held the glowing curves of childhood. Our postures held that inward-facing-ness that comes from just having stepped into the real world.

Our friendship, in many ways, held a childlike and innocent quality. In fact, our close relationship began with stories and jokes bandied over plastic lunch trays. One of the classes we took together ended just before lunch. Since we both had a break, Trent and I started going to one of the on-campus eateries together. We talked about books and the high school activities we missed. We went to college classes before and after lunch, but this was a cafeteria romance nonetheless.

As the semester continued, I found myself wanting to stand closer to him when we walked. I tried to find more excuses to be with him. I looked for him in the cafeteria at breakfast and dinner, as well as at lunch. Our cafeteria relationship extended to walks on campus, study groups, picnics with peanut butter and jelly sandwiches, and (yes, really) sing-along sessions held in a chilly tunnel on Sunday nights.

Eighteen is such a young age to be anything; it's especially young to be in love. Just three months into our friendship and budding romance, Trent volunteered to go to Argentina for a two-year religious mission. During the mission, Trent would not be able to call me, and he would have very limited access to computers. His main form of communication would be by letter.

At the time, I thought of this as a tragedy. I was eighteen, and in love. Trent would be going away for years, and it would be difficult for me to stay in contact with him. Trent left for Argentina when he was nineteen years old. When he came home, we would be twenty-one.

Twenty-one is a long time away from eighteen. If I were to pile up little markers of important life decisions made, I believe the biggest piles would be over the years eighteen, nineteen, twenty, and twenty-one. When I met Trent at age eighteen, the two of us were infant adults. When Trent returned at age twenty-one, we were mostly established selves. Instead of being the apocalypse for romance we feared, Trent's mission turned into a time of growing up that we recorded in our letters. Our letters back and forth kept us informed about the changes in each other. They also helped us to form a strong friendship that has been crucial to overcoming infertility.

It's strange to think that such a normal part of everyday life would become so crucial in our struggle. When I look back on those days, I remember running to find those letters. Every day, I would check the mailbox, sometimes up to five times a day. The letters contained no romance. Instead, we encouraged each other in our endeavors and comforted each other in our trials.

When I lost my grandfather, a nineteen-year-old Trent wrote to comfort me in my grief. When Trent wrote about his difficulties learning a foreign language mostly by immersion, I expressed my faith in his abilities. When I failed to get into the audition choir on campus, Trent expressed his faith in my voice. When Trent wrote about freezing winters and long, icy walks, I reminded him of our own long walks together in the snow. I also advised him not to fall with his hands in his pockets. When he wrote back about falling down an icy hill with his hands in his pockets, I sent him Christmas treats to nurse his bruised pride.

As we both worked our way into the real world on two separate continents, we became familiar with each other's goals and desires. We learned what caused the other frustration. We also learned what helped the other to rally.

From Trent's letters, I learned that he was laser focused, a loyal friend, and that he put the needs of others before his own. He started most of his letters talking about the people he taught and served. He shared stories about learning to catch chickens for one family and making home repairs for another. Trent never wrote about being tired, and if he wrote about frustration, it was his frustration about the limits of what he could give.

As I wrote what encouragement I could, Trent wrote to me: "Your faith and confidence in me are what help me most."

From my letters, Trent learned about my firm faith in both the religion we shared and in the goodness of people, and that we shared similar priorities. I wrote to ask about what it was like in a new country, I told him about the quirks of my teachers, and about the summers I spent working as a caregiver.

As Trent wrote me, he learned I needed reciprocal communication. After a long spell without receiving letters, I let him know: "I need a response that lets me know, without a doubt, that you are receiving my letters."

As we learned more about each other, I adjusted my writing style to make sure Trent got the support he needed, and Trent did the same for me. I made sure to fill my letters with assurances of my confidence in his abilities. He made sure that I got consistent, personal letters with responses that showed he had received and read my letters.

In our minds, we were just building our friendship. We weren't preparing for any great event in our lives. We didn't even know that, in a few short years, we would be married. We also didn't know we would be married and infertile. Now, I can clearly see that we were establishing patterns that have helped us support each other during this difficult time.

Our reactions to each other's emotional needs have reached an instinctual level. When I see that Trent is discouraged, I remind him of my confidence in him. I retell stories of the times he has made crucial and correct decisions. I remind him about what he has been able to accomplish for our family. Most of all, I remind him that I know he will be a good father and that he is already a good husband.

Without rational thought, I know he needs me to tell him that he is worthy to have children, even if he doesn't have them yet. He needs to be reminded that his hard work and study will bring about a career that will support our family. He needs to know that I see how wonderful he is to his nieces and nephews. He needs to know that I feel safer and happier because he is with me.

When Trent sees that I am discouraged, he sits me down and just has me talk to him. I explain what I'm feeling, what worries me, and what makes me afraid. He listens and lets me know he understands what I am saying. He asks clarifying questions and offers advice (unless I tell him to just listen). Sometimes, I just list back the things the doctor has told us—to make sure I understood everything.

Without rational thought, Trent knows I need my worries to be acknowledged. He knows that if I feel like I'm unnoticed or unheard, I feel cheated, aloof, and unimportant. He understands that sometimes I need an audience in order for me to compose my thoughts. He knows I need to know my feelings are intelligible or else I feel alone.

I imagine that everyone going through infertility treatment experiences a moment of complete shock. It's like getting hit by an ocean wave: you can't tell which way is up, you can't breathe, and you are powerless to come up for air. You must wait until the wave is done with you. In that moment, I'm sure it seems impossible that there is any way that you were prepared for what lies ahead. I was sure that Trent and I hadn't been. But through this trial, I've learned what I believe to be a universal truth: it isn't just the blind that are blindsided. Preparation doesn't always insulate against shock. What preparation does is allow navigation to a better state of being. Look back, and I'm sure we can all find experiences that prepared us for what we're going through.

For us, the years of friendship before our marriage prepared us as a couple. I see our preparation as vital to successfully navigating our fertility crisis. There was a time before infertility. Trent and I already existed as whole individuals with strengths and weaknesses long before this all began. We existed as a united front as well. Our tragedy has changed the means by which we have children. It did not take away our accumulated fortitude. I'm not sure why we were intended to endure this together. I assume I'll learn more about the reason in the same way I discovered that Trent and I were indeed prepared for this trial: through time and reflection. In the meantime, I can draw comfort from the fact that I was not sent into this struggle without resources.

Dear Trent,

A few days ago, we slept in. After cuddling and lounging, we had a nice brunch: pancakes, eggs, and bacon. You helped me clean up the kitchen afterwards. We didn't bother with the laundry; we went for a walk instead. It was one of the warm fall days where the sun shines with that shade of yellow that only comes when filtered through changing leaves. We even went out to dinner, a luxury in which we seldom indulge. To me, my favorite part of the day was how many hours of it we spent holding hands.

A few weeks ago, you sat preparing for another of those extensive dental school tests. The tests that require you to make flash card after flash card, hour after hour. My week also kept me busy. The dishes were piling up in the sink because I needed to meet a writing deadline. The carpets looked grubby, and the laundry spilled from the hamper, too. We needed groceries, but I couldn't go shopping because our car sat at the mechanic's shop for the fifth time this year. We were once again in that fertility limbo where we wait to see if a treatment is having any sort of effect. The word *overwhelmed* floated in the air around us like a tangible thing. When I learned I'd ordered the wrong car part online, you helped me to calm down and never mentioned the state of the apartment, nor the hours of studying you still needed to finish.

A few months ago, we went to visit my parents. We stayed a little over two weeks. With so many happy events taking place, we were distracted from the pain of our current trials. In the last two days of the trip, we went back to the hike where you proposed to me. I remembered that day with such clarity, right down to the smell of the green things growing.

A few years ago, we were coming home from the doctor's office. I don't often like to think about that day. Despite our months-long battle against infertility, until that day, we were able to cling to certain hopes. We hoped that we would only have troubles with the first pregnancy. Then, after our first success, we would get pregnant without medical intervention. We hoped that the problem could be fixed by hormone therapy or a one-time surgery. We hoped that maybe the problem would resolve in some miraculous fashion and we would never need to go to the fertility doctor again. With our new reality, our hearts were breaking right along with our shattered dreams. We spent the rest of that day crying and calling family.

About half a decade ago, I woke up at six-thirty on a cold winter morning. It was the last day I would ever wake up without you next to me. Both my mom and yours helped me get into my wedding dress. My sisters helped me with my hair and makeup. When they led me into the waiting room, you were already there. Your face projected happiness like a beacon. The clergyman gave us five minutes alone to sit and hold hands before we went into the ceremony together. Some brides get cold feet. Some grooms get butterflies. We, neither of us, doubted that we wanted to spend forever together. The next day, I woke up next to you.

Nearly a decade ago, we met at our university's welcome week. You looked distinctly Californian in your surfer shirt, jean shorts, and flip flops. I looked like I was trying too hard to be a grown up in my ballet flats, slacks, and blouse. My roommate introduced me to you, and I remember thinking you seemed nice, and you had the widest smile I'd ever seen. You tell me you remember thinking I looked pretty, and you wanted to get to know me better. It's one of the few memories I have of us walking together without either your hand in mine or your arm wrapped around my waist.

Day after day, year after year, we have so many ordinary days, so many happy times. And yet, we also have had those moments of tragedy and supreme sadness. Does everyone feel this way? Does everyone look back at the days and think, *I never knew how much joy/sadness/glory/pain was to come*? When I married you, I knew that I would be forever happy with you. The day we found out about our infertility, I thought happiness might just elude us. Infertility has taught us much about uncertainty. We've learned that so much can be taken from our control. But I think it has taught us something else, as well. It's taught us that tomorrow comes, even the day after tragedy, and that we don't need complete control in our lives to be happy in them.

There is still so much we don't know, but this much I can tell you. Tomorrow, I'm going to give you a kiss before the sun comes up. No matter what else happens, I know that I love you.

—*Emily*

Two

We were married on a post-blizzard day in December in Seattle, Washington—a place it almost never snows. The streets leading to our wedding venue were caked with grayed ice. As we traveled to Seattle from Utah, City Hall announced its imminent closure and indefinite opening time, estimated at three days after our planned wedding ceremony. As we sat on the plane, one of Trent's brothers walked from his apartment in the freezing cold to rescue our marriage license. To this day, we credit him with saving our wedding.

The ceremony lasted maybe fifteen minutes. Only family, clergy, and friends who might as well be family attended. We took few pictures after the ceremony—partly because I'd picked out my bridesmaids' outfits in summer. I didn't want them to die of cold in their short sleeves and knee-length skirts. The three-hour drive back to my hometown for the reception turned into a six-hour drive because of the snow. We made it to the reception with five minutes to spare.

At the reception, Trent and I stood in a receiving line for about three hours. I shook hands with members of my parent's church congregation, soccer coaches, high school friends, teachers, and family friends. Then we took time for another round of pictures, this time indoors with much happier bridesmaids. Trent and I didn't really eat dinner, just crammed some crab-filled pastries and chocolate mint cake down our mouths between waves of guests. Even without taking the time to eat, we arrived at our hotel at about eleven at night.

I enjoy many memories of that frenzied, wonderful, long day. Of all the many words said, hands held, and snow-caused delays encountered, one moment in particular stands out. As part of the ceremony, Trent and I had been kneeling at an altar. After exchanging our vows, the minister asked Trent to, "Please help Mrs. Adams stand." I was, quite suddenly, his wife. In a matter of a fifteen-minute ceremony, Trent and I became a family.

That was several years ago. Our family is now one person short of our expectation. In fact, we were hoping to have a second baby on the way by now. It's strange to see two- or three-year-old children and realize that, if all had gone according to plan, our child would be their age.

Like many experiencing infertility, we are a couple in limbo, a seasoned family of two. In the newlywed stage, we were still getting into the rhythm of combining our lives. We learned how to budget, how to coordinate schedules (we owned only one car), how to prepare meals for two different palettes, how to shop, how to communicate our wants and needs, even how to sleep in the same bed without elbowing each other. Learning to put a family together takes time; learning to make it run with smooth efficiency takes tremendous effort.

After about a year, we were ready to try to make adjustments for a third member of the family. Then, no third person came. Then we found the third person might take years and years to arrive. Trent and I already felt like a family, but now it was as if someone was missing. The outside world now started to see us, not as newlyweds, but as a couple. We didn't quite know what to do with that categorization. It turns out that the rest of the world can't quite categorize us either.

Almost inevitably, events planned for families are planned for families with children. I remember once seeing a storytelling event advertised at a local library. Trent and I love storytelling festivals, so we marked the date on our calendar. The event took place at a different library than the one closest to us. We got lost, and in consequence, walked in about five minutes late. Everyone watched us come in, puzzled expressions on their faces. As we made our way to our seats, I realized that all the other adults had children with them. They were looking at us, confused. We chose some seats behind a mother and her three children. She kept glancing back at us. I think she was trying to decide if our child would be coming later or if we were teenagers who came without our parents. Once, I caught her eye and smiled. She looked away, embarrassed.

We've learned to laugh it off. Some activities we've gone to held a nice mix of families with children and families without. Other times, we've shown up to find that we were expected to bring at least one child with us. Sometimes we stay at those activities. Sometimes we go home. Whichever decision we make, we try to base that decision on what would make us happy; we don't need to please anyone else.

During the holidays, Trent and I have also come to realize that most holiday activities are centered on providing a fun time for children. Decorating Easter eggs or Christmas ornaments are distinctly kid-friendly activities, for example.

In my childhood, ever since I was two years old, all the kids painted our hands and pressed them onto a quilted tree skirt. The point of this endearing ceremony is to show the growth of our family over time. When Trent and I got married, we both pressed our hands into the Christmas tree skirt, side by side. Not much visible has changed about Trent or me in the past few years. Our hands look the same as they did the day we married. At one point, we wondered why we even bothered participating.

After consideration, we decided to keep it up. The tree skirt is a record. We decided we wanted it be an accurate record of our lives. Right now, our family is staying the same size (and so are we). If I think about it, my hand stopped changing at about age fourteen, but I still pressed my hand to the tree skirt every year afterwards. It's alright to chronicle the fact that we've stopped growing, because one day, we will become a larger family. The time in between is not nothing. It's a buildup; it's an expectation. And we are a family the whole time through it.

As the world around us keeps moving, Trent and I have made the decision that we won't be left behind. And we won't be forced into a different path, either. We wanted a family-centered life, so our activities are family friendly. When Christmas comes around, we decorate our apartment, complete with a Christmas tree. We go caroling. We visit with family. We pick out a special family gift for the two of us. On New Year's Eve, we go to family parties rather than going out on the town. On St. Patrick's Day, if one of us forgets to wear green, the other is sure to pinch. We decorate Easter eggs in the spring and hide each other's Easter baskets. During Halloween, we dress up and hand out Halloween candy. At Thanksgiving, we hold family activities and play games with our nieces, nephews, cousins, and our cousin's children.

The traditions, though family-centered, will, of course, need to be adjusted when we do have children. The cookies and eggs we decorate with just the two of us are perhaps too elaborate for a young child. We will go caroling earlier in the evening when we have children and perhaps not worry about harmonizing. On Halloween, we will be escorting our own trick-or-treaters out to get candy, not staying at home handing it out. On St. Patrick's Day, we will be teaching our children the "soft-pinch" technique, and they will be informed that pinches are only for family. We don't spend our time living exactly like we would if we had children. Rather, we live as a family with no children.

It's not just at holidays that we live the family life, either. We've made adjustments in our everyday life. We decided long ago that we wanted to raise our children in the faith we grew up in. We remain active in our congregation, volunteering for tasks and accepting assignments from our minister. In addition to our weekly date, we have a special night set aside for family activities. We play games or teach lessons about religion. We make sure that no matter what activities we attend, they wouldn't be something we would be ashamed to tell our children about.

Sometimes we find ourselves in the midst of an activity where we are the only ones without children. Sometimes we forgo an activity we deem inappropriate. It might seem strange to some people the lengths we go to in order to be a family of two. But we are living the life we want, on our own terms. When our children come, we have a family life ready-built for them. We hope they love it as much as we do.

Green-Painted Docks

We jump off green-painted docks
into brown-blue water.
That's the color real lake water is,
and we have only ever been to real places.

I hear of far-off countries full of treasures:
palaces with golden doors hiding expensive foods,
plush and expensive furniture,
and all the insulation money can give
against discomfort.

We have seen those places in photos
on postcards that don't show how
even in these lands,
the streets get dusty.

There are days when we stare at the places
we've hung on our refrigerator
and eat popsicles
from the freezer
and we dream of going . . . somewhere.

But today, we are at the green-painted dock,
and we swim in the brown-blue water and feel the grit
of gravel-silt in our toes and share the lake
with the fish and ducks and mosquitos.
On shore, we munch on seeded watermelon,
and when we go home, we'll be happy.

Perfect Brightness

I've lived vibrant days
where the sun bleached the scenery almost white,
and the warmth of the afternoon baked my skin
into a comfortable, auburn tan.
There was no work to do, only light to absorb.

If I could have stayed swathed in the full comfort
of such sunbaked happiness,
and enjoyed a brightness of uninterrupted joy,
I would have leapt barefooted into that dream-world.

I would have never grown calluses on my hands
or grown wrinkles from my skin's constant change from
    pale
to rich brown—shifting with the seasons.
I would have been unfamiliar with fog, with hurricanes,
tornadoes, or snow.
And in leaving behind my pain and sorrow
for uninterrupted, constant, exhausting joy;
I'd have left each Sadness to stay where it was:
unresolved, unanswered, and unmended;
still hovering just outside the door to my paradise.
And I would have been barefoot.

All to Myself

*I*t's the nights when we make last-minute plans when I'm glad I have you all to myself. We can rush from the house at a moment's notice with no responsibilities waiting for us, no obligations until morning. After the movies, if we want to grab some hot chocolate or ice cream, we don't need to phone home. No one will worry that we are running late. If we wanted, we could spend the entire night out and about.

Sometimes, I dream about jumping in the car with you and driving until we are too tired to keep going; then sleeping in the first hotel we can find. We could if we wanted, and if we were reckless enough. Is it strange that just the thought that we could makes me smile? I look over at you and think about driving away with you, and I feel myself go warm. So I ask if we can cuddle. We sit there and hug and maybe kiss and talk. I've never yet asked you to run away with me.

Once, a group of friends invited us to go star gazing. At midnight or one o'clock, there would be a meteor shower. We grabbed some sleeping bags and drove up into the mountains with them. It was so cold, we could only keep warm by snuggling close. The sky looked clear, and the stars were as thick and white as permafrost. When the shooting stars started streaking across the sky, they looked like icicles that formed and melted in the same instant.

On lazy Saturday mornings, I love it when we wake at the same time and lay there talking underneath the covers. I feel so warm and happy. I don't care that neither my hair nor teeth are brushed. I don't care that the groceries need to be bought or that brunch needs to be fixed (because by the time we decide to get up, it will be too late for breakfast). I'm just glad to be with you.

I like that I never need to check to see if we are alone when we're at home. I never have to watch what I say. If I want to flirt with you, I can flirt to my heart's content. I can tackle you to the couch and kiss you. Never do I need to worry about being caught. We have no interruptions to worry about, no inside doors that need to be locked.

Remember that time we went to the ice rink—that student activity at our university with the hot chocolate, the cookie decorating, the broom hockey, and the mascot? It was so fun to race you around the arena—especially since neither of us was too good at stopping. We weren't allowed to form long chains with the other students, but we had a fun time trying to whip each other across the ice. Oh, how I loved it when you would skate behind me, put your hands on my hips, and push me.

The days we steal away during family vacations to visit the beach make me so happy. We go out into the waves and body surf, sometimes getting pummeled into the sand by the bigger swells. You grew up near the ocean, so finding seashells isn't all that exciting to you. Still, you help me look up and down the beach. Once, you even found me a sand dollar—a whole one. I'm not a fan of being buried in the sand—except for when you do it. You're always good about getting me out if (well, when) I start feeling claustrophobic.

Or what about the season passes to the local water park we bought? Remember how we went on all the most frightening rides? The ones you must be four feet or taller to ride? We would spend whole days just playing at the water park, going home with our skins cooked red or brown—depending on if we remembered to reapply sunscreen.

The times we've broken down on the side of the road might not be happy moments in the strictest sense of the word. I like it when you're with me, all the same. You know that I've broken down without you before. It seems so much more pleasant when you are there with me. I don't need to wait alone. I don't feel vulnerable: alone on the side of the road with a smoking car. I love that I always feel that, as long as we're together, we will be okay.

Someday, we will call the babysitter if we will be late coming home from the movies. One day, I'll know for certain that we can't run away in the middle of the night. There will be a time when we will turn down the offer to star gaze with friends. On some future Saturday, I'll make sure I'm up early enough to fix breakfast, or at least pour cereal. One day, I'll need to be more circumspect in my flirtation to you, and we'll have to remember to lock certain doors. In years to come, we'll have to hold little hands when we go to the ice rink, and we'll skate much slower. There will be a time at the water park when we will need to keep watch of those in our party who are less than four feet tall. One day, you'll find a sand dollar and give it to our baby. Someday, when we break down on the side of the road, both of us will have to reassure our kids that everything will be okay.

I look forward to the time when we get to share all these things with our children. In the meantime, I'm very glad to have you all to myself.

Today

Today was one of those rare, blessed days
with only laughter in it.
It started when I decided not to clean the toilet;
got better when you snatched
the peanut butter, jam, and bread.
By the time we arrived at the park,
we were in the rhythm of happiness:
not minding the damp spots on our knees
from the watered grass,
glorying in the wet heat as the sun climbed toward noon.
The sandwiches didn't last long,
especially after we started sharing
with the seagulls.
Was it the swing or the merry-go-round
I fell from? You tickled me so hard afterwards,
I can't remember anymore.
If you got the better of me then,
you must admit I made up for it when
we climbed the tree. I was always a fast climber.
Slides aren't as long as I remember them being,
but getting caught by you at the end
is much better than being caught by my parents ever was.
Catching you proved too much for me,
but I liked it when you kissed my bruises.
When the sprinklers came on,
we ran through them fully clothed.
On the damp drive back, we stopped at the ice cream shop
and spent the extra dollar to get shakes
instead of just scoops.
We took our treasured shakes home and
watched our favorite movie on the couch,
falling asleep in a tangled cuddle.

What did it matter that we were tired
in the morning?

PART TWELVE

FINDING HOPE BEFORE FINDING CHILDREN

Pregnancy

$\mathcal{T}$here's a time of rose-colored bliss that settles in just before marriage. During the height of that time, when I could almost smell the blooms, I started to think about how I would one day bear Trent's children. I imagined babies with Trent's nose and my eyes. I imagined toddlers with Trent's hair and my cheekbones. As I would imagine these sweet, cherubic, never-crying angels, joy swelled in my soul.

One day, in the middle of a wedding planning session, I turned to my mom and asked, "What's it like to be pregnant?"

Mom likes roses. She just isn't the type of person to pluck off the thorns, not in the literal or figurative sense. So, she gave me an honest account of her experience.

"They say you only get sick in the morning and that it only lasts for the first three months. It's not true. You can feel sick all the time, and it can last through the entire nine months. The first time you feel the baby kick, you have this magic sort of connection. You start to know who they are . . . but they can also kick things you don't want them to kick, like your kidney or your bladder. Delivery is both wonderful and awful. You are in terrible pain, but you are so excited to see that sweet little face. When the baby comes, I promise, it is all worth it and you don't regret it. I'm not gonna lie though, it hurts."

She did add that pregnancy is different for everyone, so my experience might be better. Or worse. But always incredible. With Mom's honest description, I see pregnancy as a thing of beauty, but now I can also see the trials it can bring, the thorns. It's a rose: beautiful and dangerous.

Is it strange that after so much wanting and waiting, I sometimes still feel afraid? I don't like needles. The thought of an epidural makes my spine tighten. On the other hand, I also don't like pain. The thought of delivering a child without anesthetics makes my stomach seize. I don't even try to think of what it would be like to feel nauseated for nine months with no relief.

Is it strange that after so much wanting and waiting, I sometimes feel unprepared? I want to be a mother, but despite the refiner's fire of infertility, I know I will face times of weakness. I know there will be unanticipated trials. I don't know how I will help my kids with math homework, at least not once they get past algebra. I wonder if I will be good at keeping children entertained through long car trips. Is it normal that, even though I love babies, I don't like the sound of their crying?

I explained to my husband that sometimes I felt like a kid who has stood too long at the edge of the pool. It's too late for me not to think about diving in. I've had time to assess the water temperature. I can see how deep the deepest part of the pool is.

"That's not your fault," he said.

And he's right. If we'd conceived on a normal timetable, I would have been swimming for years now. So, I revised my analogy.

"I feel like I'm on the edge of a pool, not quite ready to jump in. But it's worse than that. I feel like I have this fraying rope holding me out by my waist. I am leaning forward, trying to fall into the pool, thinking, *I'm ready. I'm ready.* Then, the rope will fray more, and I start plunging toward the water yelling, "I'm NOT ready! I'm NOT ready!" When I don't hit the water, the process starts all over again."

· He granted that was a pretty thorough description.

My fear makes me wonder if there has ever been a mother who felt ready to take her baby home and raise it to adulthood. I think of Abraham and Sarah. After nearly a hundred years of trying for children, the three divine men came. I think of how she laughed when the angels said she would have a son. Did she laugh because she didn't believe it could happen? Did she laugh for joy? Or did she laugh the hysterical laughter of someone not quite sure they can face such a miraculous responsibility?

There are times at the fertility doctor's office, when we're sitting in the waiting room, and I can't help but wonder if we are finally going to get pregnant. I imagine the rush of joy that will come from stroking the baby's peach-fuzz hair, and I worry about holding him or her properly.

I used to feel ashamed of my feelings. I worried that maybe my uncertainty caused our infertility problems. I drew some strange parallel between my own personal confidence and successful conception. If I always acted with confidence, the sperm would know which way to swim. If I felt ready to be a mother, the egg would be ready to accept the sperm. It's a silly way to think, but I believe I wanted to create a fertility problem I could fix. If the problem was only my surety, I just needed to have no fears, misgivings, or unanswered questions. Easy, right?

I can convince myself of wild things, but I can only impose on myself for so long. I know that certainty has little to do with achieving pregnancy, although having a positive attitude after fertility treatments has been shown to help. Still, I knew that I couldn't force a pregnancy just by deciding I should be pregnant.

Now, I feel rather certain that my nerves and my uncertainty are a blessing. It is one of the few instances of normalcy left to me. I must make a concerted effort to be able to have kids. It is relatively certain that I will never be surprised by a pregnancy. We will need to get extensive treatment every time we try. Despite the fact that I will need to put forth a rigorous effort to conceive, I still get to have the jitters of a first-time mother. I still get to worry about if I will be all that my children want and need. I still get to wonder if I'm ready. I have this small scrap of wonder left to me. I'll hold on to it as long and as hard as I can, until the day when I get to hold my own baby and I get to start proving myself.

Sarah

Genesis 18

I still wait for the three men to appear,
like they once appeared to Sarah.
I keep a supply of cake on my hearth,
always prepared against their coming.

In summer, I sit on the porch
in the heat of the day,
hoping the distant waves of mirage
boiling from the suburban asphalt
will settle into ancient prophet-angels.

My neighbors whisper it is past the time to hope.
The miracles of the old Middle East
hold no promise for a woman in the new world,
where they say the heavens are closed,
or perhaps were never open.
But I am Sarah, too, and angels will recognize me.

On the day the three men find me,
I know what they will say.
I know what assurance they will bring.
"Sarah shall have a son."
They said it once before;
they will say it now to me.
And if I laugh, it will not be with doubt.

Sufficient Faith

It's the pain in my stomach that wakes me.
The blood came again,
despite my hope of healing.
While lying beside my sleeping husband,
scriptures burn through my mind
of the blind seeing,
the lame walking,
and the dead rising.
I believe each miracle so deeply:
the verses feel like memories
of mud on my eyelids just before sight;
of a callused—not yet scarred—hand lifting me to my feet;
of my heart stopping, then starting at His command.
I feel the issue of blood, sticky and warm,
telling me: you are again childless.
From beneath the quilt,
I reach out my hand.
If I may but touch His robe,
I shall be made whole.
I know it.
My fingers strain toward the ragged hem
two thousand years distant.

What Is a Woman?

A can't take the concept of womanhood and put it into words alone. The definition is deeper than mere description, more solid than anatomy. The concept of motherhood, too, can't adequately be quantified. The word *mother* releases so many different sensations to my mind. There's a gender, but there's also a temperature, a scent, the sense of a physical touch on the shoulders, an age that lies somewhere between eighteen and one hundred. These two indefinable and wordless ideas of womanhood and motherhood are intrinsically linked in my mind. I think they always have been. And so, when I reached the age of twenty-four and still had no children, I started to wonder if I was a real woman.

I am not often bothered by whether or not I fit into the standard mold of womanliness. I feel comfortable marching to my own tune, which often seems to have elements of the tunes other people walk. My beat doesn't sound either stereotypical or radical. At twenty-four, I no longer worried about whether I fit someone else's definition of an ideal woman. My doubts came because I no longer fit *my own* definition of womanhood, a definition I constructed throughout most of my adolescence.

Like most children, once I hit puberty, my gender identity began to be very real and very important to me. Also like most children, my perceptions of gender differences were made up mostly from observations I made from daily life. I had no older siblings, so the teenaged young women I saw most often were girls on television.

The big attraction to becoming a teenage young woman looked, to me, as though it all revolved around going to the mall, giggling about boys, and spending hours on clothes, hair, and makeup. I much preferred hiking outdoors. I didn't care much about hair or clothes. Boys were fun to play games with. Sometimes, they were intriguing. Sometimes I thought of them as "cute," but I felt sure it was silly to just sit and giggle about them all the time. I didn't like the stereotypes I saw, and so, in reaction, I decided to try being the opposite. I tried to look and act boyish.

I chopped my hair as close to my skull as my Mom would let me. I dressed in baggy clothes in an attempt to conceal my already feminine form. To keep up with the style of times (I grew up in the 1990s), I topped my ensemble with a backward-facing hat.

When I look back at those pictures, I can't help but shake my head. My hair, so curly and thick, looked like an unkempt afro. The baggy clothes hid my figure, sure. They also made me look like I had tried to dress in my older (male) cousin's clothes. My face, though makeup-less, looked feminine. My large blue eyes, full lips, and blooming pink cheeks proclaimed my femininity to the entire world. At the time, I thought my attempts at re-making myself were foolproof. Today, I can see that rather than looking like a little tomboy, I looked like a pretty hobo girl with a bad haircut.

So I blundered through my pre- and early teen years, fighting so hard to not appear ridiculous in one way, I started looking ridiculous in another. Both my mom and dad grew concerned. They worried that I was growing too obsessed with what other people thought of me. Mom asked me about my clothing and hair choices. I told her about how I didn't like the teenage girls I saw on TV and read about in books. I told her how I even saw some of my peers try to emulate those characters. I told her I didn't like how narrow-minded and petty they seemed.

"You know," Mom said, "You don't have to be like those girls. You can act like your own kind of girl without being a tomboy."

I didn't believe her. Instead of getting frustrated with me, Mom began recommending books and movies with complex and admirable female characters. She gave me her copy of *Anne of Green Gables*. She invited me to watch Jane Austen movies with her. She even taught me the real stories behind some of the Disney princesses. It took years, but I began to soften.

One day, I asked, with just a trace of latent defiance, "Do you think I need to stop acting like a tomboy?"

"No," she said, "but I think you need to start acting like who you really are."

That hit home. I realized that for the past few years, my criteria for doing something revolved around not being "girly" rather than whether I wanted to try it. As I grew, I found I liked to hike, sing, read, write, dance, target shoot, play soccer, kick box, dress up, flirt, paint, draw, cook, and travel, and I learned that, more than anything else, I wanted to be a wife and mother when I grew up.

At eighteen, finally comfortable in my own skin, I went to college. It no longer bothered me to giggle, but I also felt no shame in playing a good game of soccer. After Trent and I married, I felt such a sense of fulfillment. I felt so feminine, so womanly, and so much like myself. My confidence reached an all-time high. Then we started trying for children.

It took a while to start to lose confidence again. When I did, this time, I hit the ground hard. No longer did I try to escape a stereotype I scorned; instead, I failed to reach an ideal I had set for myself.

It's not easy to spend so many years realizing what you want, building up an idea of what life will be like, starting to make all your decisions based on this goal, and then find out that all your preparation isn't enough. Forces of nature outside the control of either myself or my husband have thwarted what I wanted, but that doesn't make the blow any less harsh. In fact, in some ways, it feels even worse. I want to be a mother. I want to be a good woman.

These times of struggle remind me of malarial infections. There are cyclical times of normal health followed by desperate sickness. Just when it seems the fever has gone for good, another attack sets in. The difference between despair and malaria is, with malaria, the treatment is always the same. With my struggle, I've felt uplifted by several different insights. One of these came about two and a half years into our fertility crisis.

I worked from home part-time. Trent studied at school. The days started to drag as I sat at home. The money I brought in felt insignificant compared to the weight of our needs. I felt certain that my employers didn't really need me, but could replace me with ease. I sometimes felt that my creative writing would never find an audience. My melancholy sometimes made it difficult for me to settle down to a task. Trent would come home to find a dozen or so projects lying around the house—all but a few unfinished. I felt like my priority was to become a mother. Yet, I saw no significant progress toward that goal.

In frustration and despair, I told Trent, "I feel like a stay-at-home mom with no children."

Trent reminded me of me my job, and of my writing. Then, sensing that those were not enough for me, he added, "You are not a stay-at-home-mom with no children. You are a stay-at-home wife. I need you."

And there it was: Trent needed me. I already filled a laudable and essential role: wife. Though it did not take away the pang caused by the lack of children, it reminded me that I had purpose. That renewed conviction that I was necessary, even if I was only sure I was necessary to Trent, helped bolster my confidence.

The renewed conviction helped, but still I oscillate between confident and sorrowful from time to time. The thing that brings me back to a full recognition of who I am, the thing that helps me remember that I am the woman I wanted to become, is that I am still able to make a difference in the lives of children. Trent and I often spend time with our nieces and nephews. We bring them gifts every Christmas. We teach the children at our church. We babysit for our friends. When my niece confides in me, when my nephew shows me one of his drawings, when one of my church students asks me to explain a Bible passage, I see that though I am not their mother, I am important to them.

I have not yet fulfilled the peak of what I consider to be my womanly potential, but how many women reach their peak potential before thirty, anyway? Who reaches their greatest goal before they need to dye their hair? Besides, even when I have children of my own, I will need to progress more. There will be times when I need to learn to be better, so that I can help my children be better. I am not yet at my full potential, but that doesn't mean I am not a woman, nor does it mean that I will not be a mother.

Mother's Day

*A*n my home congregation, it was a tradition for the teen-agers to give all the mothers some small gift: a rose, chocolates, a potted plant, or little cards. I remember coming home to this tradition after my first year at college. I was nine-teen at the time. On Mother's Day, when the little gifts were being passed out, someone pushed an elaborate cookie into my hand.

"Oh," I said, "no, thanks. I'm not a mom yet."

I started to hand the cookie back to the young teenage boy. I guessed that he just didn't know me well enough to know I didn't have kids. My mom stopped me from handing it back. With a smile at the young boy, she ushered him away.

"They give gifts to all the women who are over eighteen and out of high school," she said.

I stared down at the cookie and felt like I had stolen some-thing.

"But I'm not a mom. I'm not married. Heck, I don't even have a boyfriend."

Mom shrugged, taking a bite from her own cookie.

"You're going to be a mother someday, though."

I still don't know why that gift of a single cookie made such an impact on me. It did, though, and Mom's explanation still didn't satisfy the nagging in my head. I've always associated motherhood with effort. Even herculean effort. I didn't feel like I held any credit towards being recognized as a mother. Mom saw the way I still stared at the frosting-covered thing with an unhappy expression.

"It's partially so that those who want to have a child but can't, or are having trouble, also get recognition."

I didn't understand. Growing up, I was used to being happy for other people's achievements, even if they achieved what I had not, and maybe would not, achieve. In my mind, I thought it would be silly for anyone to want recognition for something before achieving it. I plead youth. I plead ignorance. I plead mis-understanding.

As I said, I always equated motherhood to effort. I didn't realize the amount of effort that comes with preparing to be a parent and then in trying to conceive. I did not know that the women in the congregation who were struggling with fertility had already put forth herculean efforts for their unborn chil-dren.

Mom saw the lack of understanding on my face.

"You know, because it's not like motherhood only starts when you have children. Parenting and maternal sacrifice begin years before you have children."

I didn't get it.

"I just don't feel like I deserve it," I said.

"Well, you have it. You might as well eat it."

So I did.

In my unmarried years, I continued to feel guilty about

getting a treat on Mother's Day. I felt awkward accepting a reward for motherhood, especially when an older teenager gave it to me. I looked no older than they did, I thought.

By the time I'd reached my first Mother's Day when I knew I was having fertility troubles, the tradition had spread to the congregation Trent and I attended several states away. My aversion to the Mother's Day gift had increased exponentially. The poor people who handed me a rose never knew how much their gift tugged at my heart. I know they only meant to give a harmless gift. It's just that all I could see in that flower was failure. It was my consolation prize. If I couldn't have a baby, I could have a rose or a chocolate or a cookie.

I called home later in the day. During the call I made to wish her a happy Mother's Day, I told Mom about my own woes. She's so wonderful. Even at my most dramatic, even during the times when many would dismiss me as inconsolable or even irrational, she listens. Without blaming me, she tries to help point me in the right direction.

"It's a symbol," she said. "You are going to be a mother, aren't you?"

"Somehow. Yes. I will."

"Well, then. Why wouldn't you deserve recognition for that?"

I remember a story about Benjamin Franklin. One year, during the planting season, he decided to test the merits of using plaster as a method to help wheat grow. He poured plaster onto the wheat field, spelling out "This has been plastered." The plaster sunk into the ground, and his friends and neighbors laughed at his ideas. A week or two later, the wheat came up.

The tallest wheat with the deepest green color spelled, "This has been plastered." I feel like my mind latched on to Mom's idea in much the same way. The thought sunk deep, but took time to bloom.

It's taken years, but I think of myself as a mother now. My kids are not yet on this earth. Or if they are, they are not yet mine. But I make decisions with their welfare in mind. In fact, both Trent and I make significant decisions that will affect our children's lives. He is a father, just like I am a mother. Trent continues to pursue a career that will make enough money to support a large family, but will also allow him time off to spend at home. I work on my writing career so that I can be at home and still contribute to finances. We try to find good doctors. We keep our eyes open for good insurance coverage. Trent and I work on establishing family traditions in preparation for when our family expands. We work hard to keep our marriage healthy so that our children will come into a safe and loving home.

This past Mother's Day, as soon as the minister asked all the women to stand and receive their Mother's Day gift, I stood without hesitation. I also made sure every woman around me stood. When one of my friends sitting near me, who also suffers from infertility, expressed reluctance to stand, I motioned for her to join me.

"You might not have children yet," I said, "but you've been a mother for years."

PART THIRTEEN

REBUILDING

After the Tornado

The day after the tornado,
I found a piece of someone's
shattered dream.

I was gathering some of the debris
that cluttered the backyard—
a doll's head, soggy newspapers,
and countless shreds of plant matter—
when something sliced through my glove.

It was clear like glass,
iridescent like glitter.
Only a small shard
of an obvious masterpiece.
The tiny silver
tracings that should have
made a picture could only hint
at beauty and vastness.

I'd never seen a shattered dream before,
but how can you not
recognize someone else's
dearest wish?
Or see it for something less than it is?

Some might have tossed it right then,
thinking that to save it would be a waste,
since it is nearly
impossible to gather even
a shattered glass jug,
much less a tornado-flung fantasy.

My hand hovered over my black garbage bag,
but my fingers never opened.

If your dream is in pieces,
if it burst just in time
for the warning rush of hail
and peals of thunder,
and if you watched the fragments
of your hope become the confetti
for yet another disaster,
and you wish you knew which
of the four winds to follow first,
I live two miles east of where the tornado
touched down.

I keep a dream-shard wrapped in silk,
sitting safe at the bottom of my purse.
Even a shattered dream is worth keeping safe.

Hope

*I*n the first year of our attempts to conceive, I felt positive I would get pregnant within a few short months. Every month for about six months, I was so sure I was pregnant that I would change my eating habits: limited fish, no lunchmeats, and no soft cheeses. I even felt the symptoms of pregnancy: nausea, breast tenderness, and fatigue. But the pregnancy tests would never show up positive. A day or so after taking the test, I would start to bleed. After seven months of failed attempts, I started crying. After nine months, I started to understand that Trent and I needed medical intervention.

Still, I felt sure that we could find a successful treatment plan. I even felt rather sure that we wouldn't need to get into the more advanced treatments, like in vitro. But the months passed and passed. When we did find out the seriousness of the situation, we realized that we might never have children. That realization felt like running off a cliff when we thought we were only cresting a hill.

Of course, we still tried one of the simpler treatments. We thought it might work. We hoped it might. It didn't. As we left the doctor's office, one of the nurses called out to us. We stopped. She told us that, while we were between treatments, we should keep trying the natural way. It could still happen the natural way.

I got angry. Not at her. She was only trying to help. I got angry because I didn't want to hope anymore. I didn't want to wonder, as the month drew to a close, if I was pregnant or not. I didn't want to be disappointed again. I told her that we had been trying; we'd been trying for years. I wanted her to understand that, at this point, nature wanted nothing to do with my husband and me. I wanted her to understand that I could bear no more painful hope.

Without saying anything more, I turned and left. My husband followed. I heard the nurse try to say something more, but I was done—so done with receiving encouragement from strangers who had no idea how much it hurt to see a negative test again. I thought that hoping, even for a little longer, might just kill me.

I could have left things there and walked away from my trouble, just like I walked away from that nurse. I could have left that festering spot of disappointment alone. I could have stopped hoping and pretended I'd never wanted children. People often speak of hope like an inevitable occurrence: something as ingrained as the need to breathe. It's not.

In that moment, I looked at hope and saw perverseness instead. I could remember the nights when I went to sleep thinking, *This time. This time. This time.* I remembered waking up and wishing I needed to throw up. I remember hugging my husband close to me and feeling this half-fulfilled joy as we waited three minutes for a pregnancy test. And I remember hearing the diagnosis that meant "not this time," and realizing the nausea that was building then was just the bile of disappointment, and now I knew that unless the doctor stabbed me with needles and filled with me hormones, no pregnancy test would ever show two lines. Forever waiting on that precipice between wanting and receiving looked like a perilous hell.

When I thought of hope, I imagined myself existing poised in a space of unreality, always expecting an imminent pregnancy, sure that my prayers would be answered now. But that isn't perfect at all.

For so long, my energy, my sights, my whole soul focused on this one thing: to become a mother. I don't mean to imply I did nothing else with my life nor that I failed to strive toward other goals. Everything else just sat in the peripheral part of my mind. I could look at the other achievements in my life, my assorted potentials, combine them, and say it was not enough. Only pregnancy would be enough to make me happy.

That's not hope. Hope is about moving forward, not arriving. Pregnancy is not a destination. Neither is giving birth. Those are steps. I was looking at the world through narrowed lenses, and thought that, in order to hope, the world was suggesting I make those lenses rose colored. Perhaps it was. No matter what was suggested, what I needed was to take off those lenses and see the world entire.

I'm not quite sure what the trigger was for me. Some part of my mind believes it was that one day with the nurse. Perhaps it was the realization that I didn't want to hope that shook some part of myself loose. Perhaps it was the moment when I went in to the bookstore and realized there was nothing for me on those shelves. What I do remember was the day I started seeing a broader picture:

I was having breakfast with an author I was helping at a local writing convention. He was the keynote speaker, and I made sure he was able to get to all his events. We were talking about his current writing projects, and I told him about some of my own past projects. Then he asked me about my current ventures. I thought a moment. At that time, the main focus of my life was becoming a mother. I thought of the monumental tasks of giving my blood for tests, taking my temperature, going with my husband to doctor appointments. It took a moment to look past my self-crafted infertility lenses. I remembered a single poem I'd written about infertility. I remembered, months ago, looking at that bookshelf and despairing. I remembered finding writings on the internet, written by other women who were suffering.

"I'm writing a book about infertility," I found myself saying.

Suddenly, something else mattered, not in a peripheral way. Not that my focus had shifted from infertility to writing. No, instead my world shifted so part of my world came back from its hiding place. I looked at the world entire, instead of through the magnifying glass of my trial. I know my writing related to my struggle to become a mother. However, it was different in one key aspect: the writing could bring me no closer to having a child. With that goal that day, I started to come back to the long-forsaken world.

Living with hope bears a remarkable resemblance to just living. It's taken a while to see what the difference is, and I'm still not sure I understand the full implications of the difference. I mentioned earlier that I felt divided into two selves: Fear and Faith. Faith started as the smaller, if stronger part of me. When

I let myself hope with perfect perspective, it opened the door to Faith. Instead of being small, it is taking me over, becoming the part of me that reacts, not just reassures.

Before, each day, I struggled to defeat this problem within me, this evil that loomed over every action I took, tainted every blessing I received, and made everything I owned, felt, and knew seem insufficient. Now, I still struggle to find a solution to the problem. But the struggle is different. Letting the hope come made it possible to take action without feeling bitter. More importantly, it helped me learn that there are some days when I need to stand still and see world entire. I can accept the blessings of those days, even if the blessings have nothing to do with coming closer to having children.

And I got it. I can hope for motherhood. Even be certain of it. But I needed to understand that ways and means, dates and times, sorrows and joys, would come with methods outside of my original expectations. My life would continue forward, but not all forward movement would be toward having a child. I needed to learn to be alright, even if nothing altered in my struggle against infertility.

That's it. Hope is not about uninterrupted joy, nor is it a foolish disconnect with reality. Hope is about facing difficulty, not always knowing how it will be alright, and despite it all, living life.

Make No Mistake

No, I haven't yet borne a child.
But make no mistake,
I have children.

I often picture them
waiting at the gates
between here and heaven.
They cluster together,
their wispy spirit-bodies
barely distinguishable from
the glory behind them.

No, I haven't yet borne a child.

But I have held their images in my mind
during every doctor visit,
and tried to superimpose their faces
over the face of the crestfallen physician
as he walks into the room
with more disappointment.

I have children.

I've never met them,
but I daily plan for the needs
they will have when they come:
saving for each of their college tuitions,
learning kid-friendly recipes,
collecting picture books,
and looking for homes in nice neighborhoods.

Make no mistake.

I've loved them through every hardship and trial
with no conditions.
Not even the condition
of their presence on this earth.

No, I've never yet borne a child.
But make no mistake,
I've been a mother for years.

About the Author

*E*mily Harris Adams considers herself a long-expecting mother. She's seen the frustrating world of infertility: the often humiliating doctor visits, the astonishing price tags for treatments, having to explain why she doesn't have kids, the shock of finding out a friend is going through the same struggle, waking up with her arms cradling a non-existent baby, and needing to suddenly cancel a round of in-vitro for health concerns.

Emily is also a poet. Her first poem, *Empty Linen*, was quoted to a religious audience of more than 13 million people. Emily's award-winning poems *Second Coming* and *Birthright*. She lives in Sandy, Utah.

About Familius

Welcome to a place where mothers are celebrated, not compared. Where heart is at the center of our families, and family at the center of our homes. Where boo boos are still kissed, cake beaters are still licked, and mistakes are still okay. Welcome to a place where books—and family—are beautiful. Familius: a book publisher dedicated to helping families be happy.

Visit Our Website: www.familius.com

Our website is a different kind of place. Get inspired, read articles, discover books, watch videos, connect with our family experts, download books and apps and audiobooks, and along the way, discover how values and happy family life go together.

Join Our Family

There are lots of ways to connect with us! Subscribe to our newsletters at www.familius.com to receive uplifting daily inspiration, essays from our Pater Familius, a free ebook every month, and the first word on special discounts and Familius news.

Become an Expert

Familius authors and other established writers interested in helping families be happy are invited to join our family and contribute online content. If you have something important to say on the family, join our expert community by applying at:

www.familius.com/apply-to-become-a-familius-expert

Get Bulk Discounts

If you feel a few friends and family might benefit from what you've read, let us know and we'll be happy to provide you with quantity discounts. Simply email us at specialorders@familius.com.

Website: www.familius.com

Facebook: www.facebook.com/paterfamilius

Twitter: @familiustalk, @paterfamilius1

Pinterest: www.pinterest.com/familius

The most important work you ever do will be within the walls of your own home.

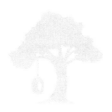

CPSIA information can be obtained
at www.ICGtesting.com
Printed in the USA
FSOW01n2108120215
5150FS

9 781939 629609